Green Home Revolution:
Eco-Friendly Hacks to Transform Your Living Space and Save Money

ISHAN ROY

Copyright Page

Copyright © 2024 All rights reserved.

No part of this book may be reproduced, stored in a retrieval system, or transmitted in any form or by any means, electronic, mechanical, photocopying, recording, or otherwise, without the prior written permission of the publisher, except for brief quotations used in reviews or scholarly works.

Disclaimer:

The information contained in this book is provided for general informational purposes only. The author and publisher make no representations or warranties with respect to the accuracy, applicability, or completeness of the content. The reader is encouraged to consult with appropriate professionals or experts before making any decisions based on the information contained in this book.

TABLE OF CONTENT

TABLE OF CONTENT...2
Introduction...5
➢ The Value of Living a Sustainable Lifestyle........ 10
Chapter 1... 19
Efficiency in Energy Use...19
➢ Natural Light and LED Lighting........................ 28
➢ Insulation and Programmable Thermostats....... 37
➢ Energy-Efficient Appliances............................... 46
Chapter 2... 55
Water Conservation: Vital Approaches for an Ecologically Sound Future... 55
➢ Low-Flow Fixtures: Improving Your Home's Water Efficiency... 65
➢ Rainwater Harvesting: An Ecological Method for Preserving Water..73
➢ **Effective Irrigation Methods: Optimising Water Utilisation for Well-Being Gardens**........................ 83
Chapter 3... 94
Sustainable Materials: Creating a More Eco-Friendly Tomorrow... 94
➢ Environmentally Friendly Building Materials: Opening the Door to Sustainable Building............ 105
➢ Low-VOC Paints: Improving Sustainability and Indoor Air Quality... 118
➢ Eco-Friendly Living Spaces: Furnishings and Décor Made of Sustainable Materials................... 129
Chapter 4...**143**

Waste Reduction: Techniques for a Future That Is More Sustainable............143
➢ Composting at Home: Using Waste to Create Priceless Resources............155
➢ Recycling & Upcycling: Creating Value Out of Waste............166
➢ Cutting Down on Single-Use Plastics: Towards a Sustainable Lifestyle............176

Chapter 5............**187**
Green Cleaning: An Eco-Friendly Way to Make Your House Healthier............**187**
➢ DIY Natural Cleaning Solutions............199
➢ Reusable Cleaning Supplies: Sustainable Home Options with Eco-Friendly Substitutes............209
➢ Eco-Friendly Brands: Leading the Way for a Sustainable Future............220

Chapter 6............**232**
Eco-Friendly Gardening: Fostering a Greener Tomorrow............**232**
➢ Organic Gardening: Using Natural Techniques to Nurture Nature............242
➢ Native and Vertical Plants: Eco-Friendly and Space-Saving Ways to Improve Your Garden............254
➢ Water-Efficient Gardening Advice: Effective Techniques for a thriving garden............263

Chapter 7............**273**
Mindful Consumption............**273**
➢ Minimalism and Ethical Shopping............283
➢ Benefits of Buying Second-Hand............293

Chapter 8............**302**

Renewable Energy: Energising the Future for Sustainability 302
➢ Solar Panels and Wind Turbines: Utilising the Power of Nature 314
➢ Geothermal Heat and Cooling: Using the Natural Energy of the Earth 324

Chapter 9 335
Green Home Design: Developing Eco-Friendly and Effective Living Environments 335
➢ Energy-Efficient Home Design: Building Sustainable and Economical Structures 346
➢ Eco-Friendly Home Renovation Tips: Using Sustainable Practices to Transform Your Space .. 356

Chapter 10 367
Living Sustainably Beyond the Home 367
➢ Eco-Friendly Transportation 377
➢ Community Involvement and Advocacy 388

Conclusion 399
Welcome to a Greener Future 399
➢ Recap of Key Points 402
➢ Encouraging Continuous Improvement 410

Introduction

The demand for sustainable living habits is more than ever in a time when environmental issues are gaining prominence in public discourse. There are many issues facing our world, such as pollution, climate change, resource depletion, and biodiversity loss. These problems pose a threat to future generations' well-being in addition to the state of our environment. It is our personal duty to change to more environmentally friendly behaviours that, when combined, can have a big influence.

This book, Green Home Revolution: Eco-Friendly Hacks to Transform Your Living Space and Save Money, will assist you on your path to a more sustainable way of living. This book offers doable, realistic tips for increasing the environmental friendliness of your house without sacrificing comfort or convenience. This book provides information and advice to assist you in making significant changes, regardless of whether you're a homeowner, tenant, do-it-yourself enthusiast, or just someone who wishes to live more sustainably.

- **The Significance of Sustainable Living**

The decisions we make on a daily basis have a significant impact on the environment. Every action we do has an impact on the ecosystem, from the energy and water we use to the things we purchase and the waste we produce. We can lessen our influence on the environment and help create a stronger, healthier ecosystem by choosing more sustainably.

In addition to preserving the environment, sustainable living also aims to improve quality of life, make living areas healthier, and even save costs. Water-saving methods, eco-friendly items, and energy-efficient housing all result in cheaper utility bills over time. Furthermore, leading a sustainable lifestyle can strengthen our bonds with the environment and promote a sense of belonging and shared responsibility.

- **The Organisation of This Book**

The eleven chapters that make up Green Home Revolution each concentrate on a distinct facet of sustainable living. The chapters are structured to be both thorough and succinct, giving you the necessary knowledge to implement real-world improvements in your house.

1. Energy Efficiency: Find out how to cut down on energy use by making easy adjustments like upgrading to LED lighting, adding insulation, and selecting energy-efficient equipment.

2. Water Conservation: Learn how to conserve water by putting in low-flow plumbing, collecting rainwater, and utilising effective irrigation systems.

3. Sustainable Materials: Examine the advantages of utilising low-VOC paints, environmentally friendly building supplies, and furniture that has been acquired responsibly.

4. Trash Reduction: Learn how to reduce trash by upcycling, composting, and recycling. You can also get advice on cutting back on single-use plastics.

5. Green Cleaning: To make your home healthier, switch to eco-friendly brands, reusable tools, and natural cleaning supplies.

6. Sustainable Gardening : Use water-saving gardening methods, select native species, and apply organic gardening practices.

7. Mindful Consumption: To lessen your impact on the environment, embrace minimalism, ethical shopping, and the advantages of buying used goods.

8. Renewable Energy: Look into alternatives for renewable energy, such as geothermal heating and cooling systems, wind turbines, and solar panels.

9. Green Home Design: Learn how to build and remodel your house to achieve the highest levels of sustainability and energy efficiency.

10. Living Sustainably Beyond the Home: Include sustainable practices in your daily activities, transportation, and community involvement.

- **Making the Initial Move**

It can be intimidating to start the transition to a more sustainable lifestyle, but it's crucial to keep in mind that every little action matters. It's not necessary to make all of the adjustments at once. Over time, progressively add more practices, starting with the ones that are most doable for you. The intention is to establish enduring behaviours that support a healthier, greener world.

This book is going to be your travelling partner, giving you the information, resources, and motivation you need to change your house and way of life. You may enhance your quality of life, save money, and have a beneficial environmental impact by using the eco-friendly tips provided in these pages.

Welcome to the Revolution of the Green Home. Together, let's take the initial step towards a future that is more sustainable.

➢ The Value of Living a Sustainable Lifestyle

More than just a fad, sustainable living is an essential strategy for protecting the resources of our world and guaranteeing a better future for everybody. It is more crucial than ever to incorporate sustainable practices into our daily lives as environmental problems like pollution, resource depletion, and climate change become more urgent. Here, we explore the main arguments for the importance of sustainable living and how it can improve our quality of life as well as the environment.

1. Taking Action to Reduce Climate Change

Climate change is one of the biggest environmental problems of our day, primarily caused by greenhouse gas emissions from human activity. Large volumes of carbon dioxide (CO_2) and other greenhouse gases are released into the atmosphere during the production of energy, transportation, deforestation, and industrial operations, all of which contribute to global warming.

We may drastically reduce our carbon footprint by implementing sustainable living practices, such as cutting back on trash, employing renewable energy sources, and reducing energy use. Climate change may be fought by taking small steps like insulating our homes, taking public transit, and buying sustainable goods. These efforts all help to lower greenhouse gas emissions.

2. Natural Resource Preservation

The natural resources of our world, such as water, minerals, and fossil fuels, are limited. Depletion, deterioration of the environment, and extinction of species are caused by overuse of these resources. In order to preserve resources for future generations, sustainable living promotes their wise usage.

Fixing leaks, installing low-flow fixtures, and utilising rainwater collecting systems are a few examples of water conservation techniques that assist in saving this essential resource. In a similar vein, we become less dependent on fossil fuels when we select energy-efficient equipment and use renewable energy sources. We also assist the preservation of forests and other natural ecosystems by purchasing products made of sustainable materials.

3. Decrease in Pollutants

Air, water, soil, noise, and other forms of pollution all pose serious risks to human health and the environment. The main causes of pollution are improper waste disposal, transportation, and industrial activity. By encouraging healthier substitutes and conscientious consumption, sustainable living approaches seek to lower pollution.

Pollutants entering our ecosystems can be significantly reduced by recycling waste, using less plastic, and switching to green cleaning products. Sustainable gardening and farming methods also reduce the need of dangerous fertilisers and pesticides, preserving the purity of the soil and water.

4. Improving Individual Health and Welfare

Personal health and well-being are strongly associated with sustainable living. We can establish a healthy living environment by lowering exposure to dangerous chemicals present in non-organic foods, personal care products, and conventional cleaning supplies. Better health results come from sustainable behaviours like using natural cleaning products, growing our own food, and consuming organic foods.

Furthermore, improved insulation and ventilation in energy-efficient dwellings lead to improved indoor air quality and a lower risk of respiratory problems. Spending time in nature and practicing sustainable gardening are two more ways to enhance general wellbeing and mental health.

5. Credit Reserves

The idea that living sustainably costs a lot of money is untrue—many eco-friendly habits can result in large cost savings. Utility costs are decreased with LED lighting, energy-efficient equipment, and adequate insulation in the home. Grocery prices can be reduced by producing your own food and using water-saving measures.

Long-term cost savings on energy costs can be achieved by making an investment in renewable energy sources, such solar panels. Purchasing used goods and upcycling materials also lessens the demand for new purchases, which results in even more cost savings.

6. Building a Community Spirit

Cooperation and community involvement are common components of sustainable living. A sense of community and shared responsibility are fostered by taking part in neighbourhood farmers' markets, community gardens, and environmental programs. Communities can build a more resilient and sustainable future by cooperating.

Advocacy and educational initiatives are also essential in raising public awareness of sustainability. We can encourage more individuals to embrace eco-friendly practices and together have a greater impact by teaching others and setting an example.

7. Building a Future That Is Sustainable

The main goal of sustainable living is to provide our children and future generations with a viable future. The world they inherit will be shaped by the choices we make today. We may leave a legacy of resilience and environmental responsibility by adopting sustainability.

Sustainable living is about making thoughtful decisions and progressively incorporating eco-friendly behaviours into our everyday routines rather than making abrupt lifestyle changes all at once. Each tiny action counts, and when taken collectively, they result in a big improvement.

One cannot stress the value of leading a sustainable lifestyle. It is crucial for preventing climate change, protecting the environment, cutting pollution, improving individual health, building community, and guaranteeing a sustainable future. We can improve the quality of life for present and future generations and create a healthy planet by embracing eco-friendly behaviours and making thoughtful decisions.

By providing you with the information and resources you need to make these adjustments, Green Home Revolution: Eco-Friendly Hacks to Transform Your Living Space and Save Money hopes to empower you.

We can set out on a path together that leads to a more satisfying and sustainable way of life.

- **Getting Around the Book**

Whether you're new to sustainable living or want to expand your knowledge, this book is meant to be easy to use and understand. You are free to read each chapter on your own, concentrating on your areas of interest. You may make adjustments at your own pace thanks to the helpful advice and detailed instructions.

- **Strengthening Transformation**

Green Home Revolution aims to equip you with the information and resources you need to make significant changes. This book will accompany you on your road towards sustainable living, offering direction, motivation, and useful tips along the way.

Set out on this path to a more economical, healthy, and environmentally friendly way of living. Together, let's transform our houses and make a positive impact on a more sustainable future.

Chapter 1

Efficiency in Energy Use

A key component of sustainable living, energy efficiency is a cost-effective way to lessen our impact on the environment. We can minimise greenhouse gas emissions, cut utility costs, and promote a more sustainable future by optimising the energy we use in our homes. This chapter examines a number of strategies for improving your home's energy efficiency, including appliances, lighting, HVAC, and overall architecture.

1. Natural Light and LED Lighting

- **Lighting with LEDs**

Making the move to LED (Light Emitting Diode) lighting is one of the easiest and most efficient ways to increase the energy efficiency of your house. Compared to conventional incandescent bulbs, LED bulbs can save up to 80% on energy costs and have a much longer lifespan of up to 25,000 hours, as opposed to merely 1,000 hours. Since they last longer, LEDs require less waste and replacements, making them an overall more environmentally friendly option.

LED bulbs not only save energy but also provide better light quality and a variety of colour temperatures to accommodate different requirements and tastes. Convenience and efficiency are enhanced by the availability of dimmable alternatives and smart versions that can be controlled remotely.

- **Light from Nature**

Making the most of natural light is another sensible way to cut back on energy use. Using daylighting, or the process of illuminating interior rooms with natural sunshine, can help minimise the demand for artificial lighting during the day. Among the techniques to improve natural light are:

- **Adding skylights or bigger windows:** This lets more light into your house.

- **Painting a room a light colour:** Light colours reflect sunlight more effectively, letting in more natural light.

- **Structurally placing mirrors:** Mirrors have the ability to reflect and intensify natural light, creating the impression of greater light and space.

You may cut down on your overall energy use by mixing energy-efficient lighting options with natural light.

2. Insulation and Programmable Thermostats

- **Thermostats with Programming**

Most of the energy used in a home is used for heating and cooling. By regulating the temperature in accordance with your schedule, a programmable thermostat can assist you in better controlling this energy use. To ensure comfort while cutting down on needless heating or cooling, you can set the thermostat, for instance, to drop while you're at work and rise before you go home.

A lot of contemporary programmable thermostats are intelligent gadgets that pick up on your preferences and make settings changes on their own. Certain ones have apps for smartphones that let you monitor and change the temperature from anywhere, even when you're not at home.

- **Warmth**

Reducing energy usage and preserving a suitable interior temperature depend on proper insulation. Your home will stay warmer in the winter and cooler in the summer thanks to insulation, which works by reducing the flow of heat between the interior and exterior of the building. Important areas to think about improving insulation are as follows:

- **Attics:** You can drastically cut down on heat loss by upgrading or adding insulation to your attic.

- **Walls:** You may lessen the strain on your heating and cooling systems by insulating your external walls to keep heat from escaping.

- **Floors and Crawl Spaces:** Insulating these areas helps keep drafts out and maintains a constant temperature within the house.

For better insulation and to stop air leaks, gaps and cracks around windows, doors, and other openings must be sealed.

3. Appliances with Low Energy Use

- Approving Appliances with Low Energy Usage

Energy-efficient appliances are made to require less energy than their traditional equivalents to accomplish the same duties. Seek out appliances bearing the ENERGY STAR® designation, as this signifies compliance with rigorous energy efficiency standards established by the Environmental Protection Agency (EPA) of the United States.

Typical Energy-Efficient Appliances Consist of:

- **Refrigerators:** By utilising improved insulation and cutting-edge cooling technologies, contemporary ENERGY STAR® refrigerators consume less energy.

- **Dishwashers:** electricity-efficient dishwashers optimise drying and wash cycles to use less water and electricity.

- **Washing Machines and Dryers:** ENERGY STAR® dryers are made to dry clothing faster and more effectively, while high-efficiency washers use less water and detergent.

- **Continuous Upkeep**

Regular maintenance is crucial to ensuring your appliances continue to run well. In order to maintain optimal appliance performance, it is recommended by the manufacturer to clean filters, coils, and other components.

4. Energy-Efficient Home Design

- **Principles of Design**

Energy-efficient house design includes the use of materials and features that cut down on energy usage right away. Among the fundamental design tenets are:

- **Orientation:** You can lessen your reliance on artificial lighting and mechanical heating and cooling by orienting your home to take advantage of natural sunshine and prevailing winds.

- **Windows Placement and Glazing:** To optimise passive solar gain and reduce heat loss, windows should be positioned strategically and energy-efficient glazing should be used.

- **Thermal Mass:** Heat is absorbed and stored by building materials having a high thermal mass, like brick or concrete, which helps to control indoor temperature and lessens the need for heating and cooling systems.

- **Efficiency Retrofitting**

Retrofitting your current house with energy-efficient features is still a feasible choice if you're not building a new house. Among the retrofitting concepts are:

The installation of energy-efficient windows and doors helps minimise heat loss and enhance insulation. Older windows and doors should be replaced with newer, more energy-efficient models.

- **Adding external shading:** Shutters, awnings, and shades can lessen solar heat gain and increase cooling effectiveness.

5. Advantages of Energy Conservation

Improving your home's energy efficiency has advantages that go beyond its effect on the environment.

- **Cost Savings:** Lower utility bills are a direct result of consuming less energy. The savings might mount up over time.

- **Increased Comfort:** A more comfortable living space is a result of better insulation, effective lighting, and efficient heating and cooling systems.

- **Environmental Impact:** Reducing your energy use can lessen your carbon footprint and help fight climate change by producing fewer greenhouse gas emissions.

- **Property Value:** Homes with higher energy efficiency ratings tend to attract more purchasers and have higher resale values.

One of the main tenets of sustainable living is energy efficiency, which has several advantages for homes and the environment. You can drastically cut your energy usage, minimise your utility costs, and contribute to a more sustainable future by implementing energy-efficient design concepts, choosing energy-efficient appliances, installing LED lighting, upgrading insulation, and employing energy-efficient appliances. Remember that every little step counts as you set out on this road to a greener house, and that when combined, these efforts can result in significant positive change.

➢ Natural Light and LED Lighting

LED Lighting and Natural Light are essential components of a home energy efficiency plan. Homeowners can drastically cut their energy use, pay less for utilities, and create a cosier living space by combining these two strategies. This is a thorough examination of how to remodel your home with LED lights and natural light.

1. The Sustainable Option of LED Lighting

- **What is LED lighting, exactly?**

Modern lighting technologies like LED (Light Emitting Diode) illumination offer a more energy-efficient replacement for conventional incandescent and fluorescent bulbs. Because LEDs are so efficient, less energy is used overall because a higher percentage of energy is converted into light rather than heat.

- **LED Lighting Benefits**

- **Electricity Efficiency:** Compared to incandescent lights, LED bulbs consume up to 80% less electricity, and compared to compact fluorescent lamps (CFLs), they use between 30% and 50% less energy. Lower electricity costs and a smaller environmental effect are the outcomes of this efficiency.

- **Longevity:** Compared to conventional lights, LEDs have a far longer lifespan. LEDs can last up to 25,000 hours or longer, whereas incandescent lights last roughly 1,000 hours and CFLs last about 8,000 hours. Because of its lifetime, there will be less waste and replacements.

- **Reduced Heat Output:** LEDs generate very little heat, in contrast to incandescent bulbs, which release a large amount of heat. During the warmer months, this decrease in heat output may also result in cheaper cooling expenses.

- **Greater Light Quality****: With a variety of colour temperatures, from warm white to cold daylight, LEDs provide greater light quality. They offer steady, flicker-free illumination and come in dimmer choices to accommodate different lighting requirements.

- **Smart Features:** A lot of contemporary LEDs have smart features like timers, remote controls, and home automation system compatibility. Personalised lighting experiences and increased energy savings are made possible by this extra convenience.

- **Putting LED Lighting in Place**

- Replace Existing Bulbs: In high-traffic areas such as living rooms, kitchens, and restrooms, begin by swapping out incandescent and CFL bulbs with LED substitutes.

- Use LED Fixtures: To maximise energy savings and preserve a contemporary look, think about adding LED fixtures and recessed lighting.

- Select Intelligent LEDs: Use voice commands or smartphone apps to operate lighting systems and smart LED bulbs, which will enable more accurate lighting management.

2. Making the Most of Natural Light

- **The Advantages of Natural Lighting**

Daylight, often known as natural light, is a free and plentiful source of lighting that can drastically lower the demand for artificial lighting. Making efficient use of natural light has the following advantages:

- Reduced Energy Consumption: You can cut down on artificial lighting by utilising daylight as much of the day as possible. This lowers power use and energy costs.

- Enhanced Mood and Productivity: Research has demonstrated that exposure to natural light enhances mood, boosts output, and fosters general wellbeing. Better sleep patterns can result from natural light's ability to control circadian rhythms.

- Improved Indoor Environment: Daylight makes interior rooms feel more open and airy and makes them feel more pleasant and inviting.

- **Tips for Getting the Most Out of Natural Light**

- Window Placement and Design: Arrange windows so that they receive as much natural light as possible.

Throughout the day, windows facing south usually get the most sunlight. To enhance daylight penetration, think about installing skylights or utilising larger windows.

- **Light-Colored Interiors:** To reflect and enhance natural light and give the impression that a room is larger and brighter, paint the walls and ceilings in light colours.

- **Reflecting Surfaces:** To improve how natural light is distributed throughout a space, include mirrors and reflecting surfaces in your interior design.

- **Window Treatments:** Select coverings that provide adjustable control over the amount of natural light coming in. Sheer curtains and movable blinds are two solutions that can assist control sunlight while preserving privacy.

- **Harmonising Artificial and Natural Lighting**

Even though natural light is often preferable, there are occasions when artificial lighting is required, particularly on overcast days or nights. To maximise comfort and energy efficiency, the aim is to balance natural and artificial light:

- **Layered Lighting:** To create a well-lit and adaptable room, combine natural light with several artificial lighting options, such as ambient, task, and accent lighting.

- **Automatic Controls:** To ensure economical use of electricity, artificial lighting can be adjusted based on the availability of natural light by using daylight sensors and automatic dimmers.

- **Continuous Upkeep:** Maintaining clear and unobstructed windows will optimise the quantity of natural light that enters your house.

3. Integrating Natural and LED Lighting

Your home's lighting system operates more effectively and efficiently overall when LED lighting is combined with natural light. Here's how to successfully mix the two:

- Daylight Harvesting: Install LED lights equipped with daylight sensors, which change their brightness according to the quantity of available natural light. This guarantees the use of artificial lights only when required.

- Task Lighting: During the day, use natural light for overall illumination and use LED task lights for areas like workspaces where focused illumination is required.

- Circadian Lighting: To promote circadian rhythms and improve wellbeing all day, think about utilising LED lights that replicate the patterns of natural daylight.

Natural light and LED lighting are essential for improving energy efficiency and establishing a cosy living space. Adopting LED lighting technology and making the most of natural light will help you save a lot of energy, lessen your impact on the environment, and enhance the quality of your indoor areas.

Putting these tactics into practice helps you live a more sustainable lifestyle in addition to saving money. By implementing these adjustments, you'll be able to lower the energy usage of your house and make it a more environmentally friendly place to live.

➢ Insulation and Programmable Thermostats

Two essential elements of energy efficiency in the home are programmable thermostats and effective insulation. Together, these components maximise heating and cooling, save energy use, and improve comfort levels. This section examines the advantages of programmable thermostats, the significance of adequate insulation, and useful implementation advice.

1. Intelligent Climate Management with Programmable Thermostats

With the help of a programmable thermostat, homeowners can establish distinct temperatures for different times of the day and days of the week. You may save energy when you're not home or when you're sleeping by setting your thermostat to change the temperature according to your schedule, all without compromising comfort.

- **Advantages of Thermostatic Programming**

- **Energy Savings:** By automatically altering temperatures during periods of inactivity, programmable thermostats can assist lower heating and cooling expenses. For instance, you can save energy waste by turning up the temperature before you leave for work or turning it down when you get home.

- **Enhanced Comfort:** You may keep a comfortable indoor climate when you're at home and asleep by scheduling the thermostat to coincide with your routine. Over time, smart thermostats are able to learn your preferences and change the settings accordingly.

- **Convenience:** You can remotely adjust the temperature of your house with many contemporary programmable thermostats thanks to their Wi-Fi connectivity and smartphone apps. Flexibility and convenience are offered by this function, particularly in the event that your plans alter or you wish to update settings while you're abroad.

- **Integration with Smart Home Systems:** To establish a unified and automated climate management system, programmable thermostats can frequently be combined with other smart home appliances, like voice assistants and smart sensors.

- Calculated Thermostat Types

- **7-Day Programmable Thermostats:** Perfect for homes with diverse schedules, these thermostats allow you to set the temperature differently every day of the week.

- **5-2 Programmable Thermostats:** Ideal for people with regular work and play schedules, these thermostats have distinct settings for the weekdays and the weekends.

- **Smart Thermostats:** Equipped with cutting-edge features including remote access, learning algorithms, and home automation system integration.

- **Setting Up and Operating a Thermostat with Programmability**

- **Placement:** To achieve accurate temperature readings, install the thermostat in the centre of the room, away from drafts, direct sunshine, and heat sources.

- **Scripting:** Adjust the thermostat to suit your weekly and daily schedule. To optimise energy savings, incorporate temperature adjustments for periods when you're asleep or away.

- **Regular Updates:** Adjust the thermostat settings on a regular basis to account for schedule or preference changes.

2. Insulation: Preserving Comfort

- **Definition of Insulation**

A substance called insulation is used to lessen the amount of heat that is transferred from a building's exterior to inside. Maintaining a constant interior temperature lowers the need for excessive heating or cooling, increasing energy efficiency. This is made possible by proper insulation.

- **Insulation Types**

- **Fibreglass:** Often applied as a blanket or batt, fibreglass insulation works well to insulate floors, walls, and attics. It is reasonably priced and has strong heat resistance.

- **Foam Board:** Insulating walls, roofs, and foundations with rigid foam board offers excellent thermal resistance. It works well in places that are prone to wetness and is resistant to moisture.

- **Spray Foam:** By filling in cracks and spaces, expanding spray foam insulation forms an airtight seal. It works very well for air sealing as well as thermal insulation.

- **Cellulose:** This environmentally friendly insulation has good thermal performance and is made from recycled paper products. Usually, it is applied to walls and attics as insulation.

- **Advantages of Adequate Insulation**

- **Energy Savings:** By minimising heat gain in the summer and heat loss in the winter, effective insulation lowers the demand for heating and cooling. Lower energy costs and increased overall energy efficiency are the results of this.

- **Enhanced Comfort:** By eliminating drafts and cold areas, adequate insulation contributes to the maintenance of a constant interior temperature. This enhances the comfort of one's living space.

- **Noise Reduction:** Insulation also contributes to a quieter interior environment by reducing outside and inter-room sound transmission.

- **Environmental Impact:** Insulation helps reduce greenhouse gas emissions and promotes a more sustainable lifestyle by consuming less energy.

- **The Insulation Area**

- **Attics:** Improving or adding insulation in the attic lowers heat loss through the roof, making it one of the best methods to increase house energy efficiency.

- **Walls:** Insulating external walls can enhance thermal comfort and stop heat loss. Retrofitting or new construction can accomplish this.

- **Flooring and Crawl Spaces:** Insulating flooring is a good way to keep a pleasant interior temperature and stop heat loss, especially if the floors are above unheated areas like garages or crawl spaces.

- **Installing and Keeping Insulation in Place**

- **Assessment:** Determine what sections in your house need to be improved and assess the insulation levels at the moment. Enhancing insulation and identifying heat-loss spots can be accomplished with the use of an energy audit.

- **Installation:** When installing insulation, adhere to manufacturer guidelines and industry best practices. Achieving the required performance and energy efficiency requires proper installation.

- **Maintenance:** Check insulation periodically for indications of settling, dampness, or damage. Resolve any problems as soon as possible to keep performance at its best.

3. Combining Insulation and Programmable Thermostats

Programmable thermostats and efficient insulation work together to provide a holistic approach to energy efficiency:

- **Optimised Climate Control:** Adjust temperature settings according to insulation performance using programmable thermostats. For example, you can set the thermostat to benefit from the insulation's capacity to keep the temperature steady if your house is well-insulated.

- **Reduced Heating and Cooling Demands:** Insulating your home properly lessens the strain on your HVAC systems. This enhances the efficiency of programmable thermostats, resulting in more energy savings and better comfort.

- **Steady Comfort:** Maintaining a steady indoor environment improves overall comfort and energy efficiency. This is achieved via the use of intelligent temperature management in conjunction with appropriate insulation.

Effective insulation and programmable thermostats are useful resources for creating a more pleasant and energy-efficient house. You may contribute to a more sustainable living environment, cut utility costs, and consume less energy by implementing these technologies.

Adopting programmable thermostats makes it possible to precisely regulate the temperature in your house, and having enough insulation guarantees that your HVAC systems run well. When combined, these components improve comfort and energy efficiency in a synergistic way. You'll be moving in the right direction towards a more economical and environmentally friendly home as you put these tips into practice.

➢ Energy-Efficient Appliances

Energy-efficient appliances are made to operate at the same level as conventional appliances but with reduced energy consumption. Homeowners may minimise their environmental effect, lower electricity bills, and consume less energy by selecting energy-efficient appliances. The advantages of energy-efficient appliances, important characteristics to look for, and useful advice for incorporating them into your house are all covered in this section.

1. What are appliances that use less energy?

Appliances that have been built to use the least amount of energy possible without sacrificing functioning are known as energy-efficient appliances. These gadgets frequently fulfil energy efficiency requirements that are specified by independent or governmental bodies. Refrigerators, washing machines, dishwashers, and air conditioning and heating systems are typical examples.

Energy-Efficient Appliance Benefits

- **Limited Energy Use:** Cutting-edge technology is used by energy-efficient appliances to reduce energy use. This results in reduced energy costs and less stress on the power supply in your house.

- Environmental Impact: These appliances lessen greenhouse gas emissions and the need for energy production from non-renewable sources by using less energy.

- Cost Savings: While the initial cost of energy-efficient appliances may be greater, over time, these costs can be compensated by the reduction in energy bills. Rebates and other incentives are frequently offered with energy-efficient appliances, significantly lowering their initial prices.

- Enhanced Performance: Compared to previous models, contemporary energy-efficient appliances operate better and are more convenient since they frequently have cutting-edge features and upgraded technology.

2. Important Elements to Consider

The following qualities and certifications should be taken into account while looking for energy-efficient appliances to make sure you're selecting items that adhere to strict performance and efficiency requirements:

- **Energy Star Certification:** Products bearing the Energy Star mark are known for their energy efficiency. Appliances certified by this body adhere to strict energy efficiency standards established by the Environmental Protection Agency (EPA) in the United States or comparable agencies in other nations. Appliances that have undergone testing and verification for their ability to save energy can be easily identified by looking for the Energy Star label.

- **Annual Energy Consumption:** To find out the appliance's annual energy consumption, look for the energy guide label. This label lets you compare the efficiency of several models by giving you an approximate idea of how much energy the appliance will use in a year.

- **Smart Technology:** A lot of energy-efficient appliances are now outfitted with smart technology, which lets you utilise home automation systems or smartphone apps to monitor and manage your energy usage. Energy efficiency can be further maximised with features like remote control, programmable settings, and energy usage tracking.

- **Advanced Features:** Seek out appliances with energy-saving features including eco-friendly drying and washing cycles, energy-efficient compressors, and variable speed motors. These functions contribute to preserving performance while consuming less energy.

3. Different Kinds of Energy-Saving Appliances

- **Cold Storage Units**

- **Technology:** To reduce energy consumption, modern freezers feature LED illumination, improved insulation, and energy-efficient compressors. Efficiency can be further increased with models that have energy-saving modes and tunable temperature controls.

- Size and Design: Since larger refrigerators use more energy, pick a size that meets your demands without taking up too much room. French door or bottom freezer versions are usually less efficient than top-freezer models and side-by-side designs.

- **Cleaning Equipment**

- Front-load vs. Top-load: In general, front-load washers use less energy than top-loading ones. Because of their rapid spin speeds, which extract more water and cut down on drying time, they require less water and detergent.

- Features That Conserve Energy: Seek for washing machines with high efficiency settings, eco-friendly wash cycles, and water level adjustments. Additionally, certain versions have intelligent functions for monitoring and remote control.

- **Loafers**

- **Efficiency:** Dishwashers with reduced electricity and water consumption per load are energy-efficient. Frequently, they come equipped with soil sensors, movable racks, and environmentally friendly washing cycles that maximise efficiency while preserving resources.

- **Noise Level:** Energy-efficient dishwashers of today are made to run silently, improving the comfort of your house without compromising functionality.

- **Systems of Heating and Cooling**

- **Heat Pumps:** Capable of providing both heating and cooling, heat pumps are extremely effective systems. As opposed to producing heat, they function by transferring it, which uses less energy than conventional systems.

- **High-Efficiency HVAC equipment:** Seek HVAC equipment with high heating and cooling annual fuel utilisation efficiency (AFUE) ratings as well as high seasonal energy efficiency ratios (SEER). Higher efficiency and cost reductions are indicated by these grades.

- **Heating Water**

- **Tankless Water Heaters:** By only heating water when needed, tankless (or on-demand) water heaters cut down on the standby energy losses connected with conventional tank-style heaters.

- **Heat Pump Water Heaters:** These systems offer significant energy savings over traditional electric water heaters by transferring heat from the air to the water using heat pump technology.

4. Guidance on Including Energy-Saving Appliances

- **Perform an Energy Audit:** Assess your existing appliances and determine which ones use less energy.

Finding the places where improvements can have the most effects can be aided by an energy audit.

- Prioritise Upgrades: Give top priority to swapping out the most energy-hungry appliances initially. HVAC systems, washing machines, and refrigerators frequently have the biggest effects on energy usage.

- Utilise Rebates and Incentives: Buying energy-efficient appliances can result in rebates or incentives from a number of utilities and government initiatives. Look into local initiatives that can help lower the cost of improvements.

- Maintain Appliances: Energy-efficient appliances can operate better and last longer with regular maintenance and correct use. When it comes to maintaining, cleaning, and using your appliances, heed the manufacturer's instructions.

A cost-efficient and sustainable home must have energy-efficient appliances. Homeowners can experience significant energy savings, lower electricity costs, and a smaller environmental impact by choosing and integrating these products. Adopting energy-efficient technologies helps the environment and your pocketbook at the same time.

Think about each product's sophisticated features, certifications, and long-term advantages when selecting energy-efficient appliances. You may lower your energy usage, improve the comfort of your home, and contribute to a cleaner future by making wise decisions and placing a high priority on energy efficiency.

Chapter 2

Water Conservation: Vital Approaches for an Ecologically Sound Future

Water conservation is a fundamental part of sustainable living and a must for protecting the most important resource on Earth. Water efficiency and waste reduction are more important than ever due to growing population, climate change, and environmental deterioration. This section examines the value of water conservation, doable home conservation techniques, and the larger effects of these initiatives on the neighbourhood and environment.

1. Water Conservation's Significance

- **The Significance of Water Conservation**

All life depends on water, which is also necessary for industry, agriculture, and daily human activities. Fresh water, however, is a limited resource; just a small portion of Earth's water is accessible and fresh. Water shortage is becoming a worry as a result of population increase and economic development increasing the demand for water.

- **Impact on the Environment**

- Ecosystem Health: By guaranteeing that rivers, lakes, and wetlands have sufficient water levels to support plant and animal life, water conservation contributes to the upkeep of healthy ecosystems.

- Climate Change: By lowering the energy needed for transportation and water treatment, as well as by lowering greenhouse gas emissions, reducing water usage can help lessen the consequences of climate change.

- Resource Management: By conserving water, we can lessen the demand on our water supply and improve resource management, which will guarantee that our children and grandchildren have access to clean water.

- **Financial Gains**

- **Cost Savings:** Cutting back on water use results in lower utility costs and a reduction in the demand for pricey water infrastructure upgrades. The energy needed to heat and purify water can be decreased by using water efficiently.

- **Increased Property Value:** Water-saving solutions can raise the value of homes and businesses and make them more appealing to buyers who care about the environment.

2. Doable Home Water Conservation Techniques

- **Water Conservation Indoors**

- **Fix Leaks:** Water waste can occur from leaky pipes, toilets, and faucets. Keep an eye out for leaks and fix them right away. Hundreds of gallons of water can be wasted annually by a single leaky tap.

- **Install Water-Efficient Fixtures:** Replace your old fixtures with water-saving models, like dual-flush toilets, faucets, and showerheads. These fixtures function just as well while using less water.

- **Efficient Showering:** Use a water-saving showerhead and set a duration limit of 5 to 10 minutes for your showers. Showering for shorter periods of time saves electricity and water.

- **Full Loads Only:** Only operate washers and dishwashers when there are completely full loads. Modern appliances are more efficient when used to their full potential even if many of them are made to use less water each load.

- **Switch Off the Tap:** Make sure not to run the water when shaving, cleaning your teeth, or washing your hands. While cleaning, turn off the tap and just turn it back on as needed.

- **Reducing Water Outside**

- **Watering Wisely:** To minimise evaporation, water plants and lawns in the early morning or late evening. The best way to get water to the roots of your plants is to use soaker hoses or a drip irrigation system.

- **Select Drought-Tolerant Plants:** While designing a landscape, opt for native plants that can withstand drought. These plants need less water, fertiliser, and pesticides because they are acclimated to the climate in the area.

- **Mulch:** To conserve soil moisture and lessen the need for regular watering, apply mulch around plants and garden beds. Mulch enhances the condition of the soil and aids with weed control.

- **Rain Barrels:** Use rain barrels to catch and store rainfall for gardening and plant watering. This lessens erosion and stormwater runoff in addition to conserving tap water.

- **Technological Innovations**

- **Smart Irrigation Systems:** Make use of intelligent irrigation controllers that modify watering schedules in response to plant requirements, soil moisture content, and meteorological circumstances. These solutions aid in waste reduction and water optimisation.

- **Graywater Recycling:** Install systems for recycling graywater to repurpose water from showers, sinks, and washing machines for flushing toilets and irrigation in non-potable uses.

3. Water Conservation's Wider Effects

- **Community Advantages**

- **Reduced Pressure on Water Supply:** Especially in regions that are facing drought conditions, community-wide water conservation initiatives can lessen the burden on nearby water supplies and lower the likelihood of shortages.

- **Improved Water Quality:** Conservation measures can help rivers, lakes, and reservoirs have improved water quality by lowering runoff and minimising the need for unnecessary water treatment.

- **Enhanced Resilience:** Communities that conserve water are more resilient overall and sustainable since they are better prepared to withstand extreme weather conditions and variations in water availability.

- **International Viewpoint**

- **Addressing Water Scarcity:** Global water resources can benefit from water conservation measures implemented in one area. Water scarcity issues are addressed and fair access to clean water is supported globally through efficient water use.

- **Promoting Sustainable Development:** One of the main objectives of the Sustainable Development Goals (SDGs) established by the UN is water conservation. Individuals and communities can support larger initiatives to accomplish these objectives and advance environmental sustainability by practicing water conservation.

4. Overcoming Obstacles and Promoting Acceptance

- **Difficulties**

- **Education and Awareness:** A lot of people don't realise how much water is wasted or how crucial it is to conserve water. It is crucial to educate and raise awareness among the general people about efficient conservation techniques.

- **Behavioural Change:** It can be difficult for some people to make the daily routine and behaviour changes necessary to implement water-saving measures. It is frequently necessary to overcome resistance to change in order to promote the adoption of conservation techniques.

- **Promoting Acceptance**

- **Incentives and Rebates:** Water-efficient fixtures and appliances may be eligible for incentives and rebates from governments and utilities. These monetary rewards can aid in defraying upfront expenses and promote a wider adoption rate.

- **Community Programs:** Take part in neighbourhood seminars, school programs, and local campaigns, among other community activities and initiatives, that encourage water saving. Together, we can make a bigger difference and promote a conservation mindset.

- **Personal Accountability:** Establish goals for your household and yourself to conserve water, monitor your progress, and acknowledge your successes. Setting a good example and sharing accomplishments encourage others to follow suit.

One of the most important components of sustainable living that helps communities, the economy, and the environment is **water conservation**. People may help ensure that this priceless resource is preserved and available for future generations by adopting doable water-saving techniques at home and by supporting larger conservation initiatives.

For the globe to become more resilient and sustainable, it is imperative that people recognise the value of water conservation and take concrete measures to cut back on their usage. Each action you take to create a more environmentally friendly and water-conscious future—from plugging leaks and installing energy-efficient fixtures to embracing cutting-edge technology and becoming involved in neighbourhood projects—matters. Adopting water-saving techniques not only contributes to environmental protection but also encourages a more conscientious and sustainable lifestyle.

➢ Low-Flow Fixtures: Improving Your Home's Water Efficiency

Low-flow fixtures, which are made to drastically cut water usage without sacrificing functionality, are a crucial part of water conservation initiatives. These fixtures have a significant positive influence on the environment and save a lot of money on utility bills because they are very good at controlling household water consumption. This section examines low-flow fixture types, installation, and benefits, providing helpful advice on how to incorporate them into your house.

1. Gaining Knowledge About Low-Flow Fixtures

- **What Are Fixtures With Low Flow?**

Plumbing fixtures known as low-flow fixtures are made to consume less water than conventional fixtures without sacrificing or improving functionality. They do this by utilising cutting-edge technology that controls water flow to reduce waste. Typical examples of low-flow fixtures are faucets, toilets, and showerheads.

Advantages:

- **Water Conservation:** Low-flow fixtures contribute to a reduction in total water usage, which is important in regions that are facing drought or water scarcity. These fixtures help ensure the sustainable management of water resources by consuming less water.

- **Cost Savings:** Lower water bills result from less water use. Furthermore, a lot of low-flow fixtures include energy-efficient designs, which reduces the energy used to heat water even more.

- **Environmental Impact:** Low-flow fixtures contribute to lessening the load on water treatment facilities and the energy needed for water heating and pumping by using less water. This lessens the impact of water use on the environment.

2. Low-Flow Fixture Types

- **Showerheads with Low Flow**

- **Technology:** Low-flow showerheads lower water flow without sacrificing water pressure by utilising a variety of technologies. Aerating shower heads, which combine air and water to produce a more intense spray, and laminar-flow showerheads, which produce a smooth, unaerated stream, are examples of common designs.

- **Flow Rate:** 2.5 gallons per minute (GPM) is the typical flow rate of traditional shower heads. With their 1.5 to 2.0 GPM flow rates, low-flow devices can drastically cut water use without sacrificing the enjoyment of a pleasant shower.

- **Installation:** There is no need for specific tools for the simple installation of a low-flow showerhead. Just remove the current showerhead and swap it out for the low-flow type. Make sure it fits snugly and look for leaks.

- **Small-Flow Taps**

- **Technology:** Aerators or flow restrictors are used by low-flow faucets to lower water flow. While flow restrictors regulate the volume of water that comes out of the tap, aerators combine water and air to produce a continuous, level stream.

- **Flow Rate:** The typical flow rate of a tap is 2.2 GPM. With flow rates of 1.5 to 2.0 GPM, low-flow faucets provide a notable reduction in water use without compromising performance.

- **Installation:** Installing low-flow faucet aerators is simple; just screw them onto the current faucet. For more extensive improvements, think about switching out the entire tap for a low-flow variant.

- **Low-Flow Plumbing**

- **Technology:** Compared to conventional versions, low-flow toilets consume less water per flush. They frequently include dual-flush systems, which further reduce water usage by providing distinct flush choices for liquid and solid waste.

- Flush Volume: A typical flush on a traditional toilet uses between 3.5 and 7 gallons. Low-flow toilets drastically cut down on water usage, using between 1.28 and 1.6 gallons every flush.

- Installation: To install a low-flow toilet, take out the old one and install the new one. For optimum efficiency and to prevent leaks, make sure the installation is done correctly.

3. Selecting and Fitting Low-Flow Appliances

- **Choosing the Appropriate Fixture**

- Take Flow Rates into Consideration: Make sure the low-flow fixtures you choose match your needs by comparing flow rates. Seek out fixtures bearing the WaterSense logo, since it signifies their compliance with stringent water efficiency and performance standards.

- **Evaluate Performance:** Check fixtures for proper performance and water pressure. Low flow does not always equate to poor performance; many contemporary fixtures provide better functionality and user experiences.

- **Installation Advice**

- **DIY Installation:** A lot of low-flow fixtures are made to be installed simply, and even homeowners with rudimentary plumbing knowledge may accomplish this. To stop leaks, make sure the fitting is tight and adhere to the manufacturer's instructions.

- **Expert Installation:** You should think about contacting a professional plumber for more intricate installations, such as replacing a tap or installing low-flow toilets. Appropriate setup and functionality are ensured by professional installation.

4. Keeping Low-Flow Fixtures in Working Order

- **Continuous Upkeep**

- **Clean Aerators and Showerheads:** Mineral deposits can accumulate in aerators and showerheads over time, reducing their functionality. Keep these parts clean on a regular basis to provide the best possible water flow and efficiency.

- **Inspect for Spills:** Check fixtures for drips or leaks on a regular basis. Resolve any problems as soon as possible to save water waste and preserve fixture functionality.

- **Optimisation of Performance**

- **Adjust Flow Rates:** Adjustable flow rates are possible with some low-flow fittings. To modify the flow if it's too high or too low, see the manufacturer's instructions.

- **Upgrade Components:** To increase water flow and efficiency, think about upgrading components like aerators or flow restrictors if performance problems occur.

Low-flow fixtures are an important component of water conservation initiatives, providing a number of advantages in terms of water conservation, financial savings, and environmental effect. Homeowners can significantly contribute to sustainable living and resource management by selecting and installing low-flow showerheads, faucets, and toilets.

Using low-flow fixtures is a sensible and efficient approach to cut water usage without sacrificing comfort or performance. Every attempt to improve water efficiency contributes to a more sustainable future and helps protect this essential resource for future generations, whether through straightforward improvements or significant adjustments.

➤ Rainwater Harvesting: An Ecological Method for Preserving Water

Rainfall harvesting is a novel and environmentally friendly technique that includes collecting and holding onto rainfall for a variety of applications, including gardening, irrigation, and even drinking water. By collecting water in this way, you can lessen your need on municipal supplies, save money on utilities, and protect the environment. The fundamentals of rainwater harvesting, its advantages, different systems and techniques, and useful tips for installing a system at home are all covered in this part.

1. Gaining Knowledge About Rainwater Harvesting

- **What is Harvesting Rainwater?**

The technique of gathering and storing rainwater from roofs, sidewalks, or other surfaces for later use is known as rainwater harvesting. Rainwater collection can be filtered and treated to suit individual requirements, from irrigation and other non-potable applications to potable uses following appropriate treatment.

- **Evolution and History**

The idea of collecting rainwater is not new. It has been used for thousands of years in many areas and cultures. Rainwater collection systems were employed for home and agricultural uses by ancient civilisations, including the Greeks, Romans, and Chinese. These systems have been improved by recent developments, which have integrated technology and increased efficiency to match modern demands.

2. Advantages of Collecting Rainwater

- **Detrimental Effects**

- **Water Conservation:** Households can lessen their reliance on municipal water supplies and help preserve local water resources by collecting and using rainwater.

- **Decrease in Stormwater Runoff:** Rainwater collection contributes to a reduction in stormwater runoff, which lessens the strain on stormwater management systems, prevents flooding, and lessens erosion.

- **Sustainable Use:** Harvested rainwater has a smaller environmental impact since it requires less energy for transportation and water treatment.

- **Financial Gains**

- **Cost Savings:** Water bills can be significantly reduced by reducing dependency on municipal water. Rainwater collection can also be utilised for landscaping and irrigation, negating the requirement for expensive municipal water for these uses.

- **Increased Property Value:** The extra sustainability features and potential savings on utility bills associated with rainwater harvesting systems may make a property more valuable.

- **Utilitarian Advantages**

- **Reliability:** Rainwater collection offers an extra, dependable source of water in regions vulnerable to drought or water constraint.

- **Versatility:** Reclaimed rainwater can be utilised for a variety of tasks, such as washing clothing, watering gardens, flushing toilets, and, with the right preparation, producing drinking water.

3. Categories of Systems for Harvesting Rainwater

1. Rainwater harvesting on rooftops

- **System Components:** This system gathers rainfall from the roof, directs it down downspouts and gutters, and stores it in cisterns or tanks. Usually, the system has filters to keep things clean and free of debris.

- **Advantages:** Rooftop harvesting is a very efficient way to collect a lot of water, and it fits in well with existing buildings.

- **Points to Ponder:** To preserve the quality of the water, make sure that the roofing materials and the gutters are clean and clear of pollutants.

2. The Harvesting of Surface Rainwater

- **System Components:** This technique gathers rainfall from parking lots and driveways, among other paved and unpaved areas. Water is preserved for later use by being diverted into ponds or collection basins.

- **Advantages:** It can enhance water capture when combined with rooftop systems.

- **Considerations:** Because surface water contains more impurities, it might need more thorough filtering and treatment.

3. Rainwater Harvesting Below Ground

- **System Components:** Rainwater is diverted into subterranean storage tanks or cisterns after being gathered from various surfaces. To guarantee water quality, these systems frequently include filtration and treatment units.

- **Advantages:** Compared to above-ground tanks, underground systems are less noticeable and help conserve space.

- **Considerations:** Because of the needs for excavation and building, installation may be more complicated and expensive.

4. Putting a Rain Harvesting System in Place

- **Organisation and Layout**

- **Assess Water Needs:** Find out how much water is necessary for different purposes as well as how big of a rainwater harvesting system is needed.

- **Assess Site Situation:** To create an effective system, consider the size, surface area, and local rainfall patterns of the roof. Take into account elements like the type of roof and any possible pollutants.

- **Choose Elements:** Select the right parts, such as pumps, storage tanks, filters, gutters, and downspouts. Make sure every material is strong and appropriate for collecting rainwater.

- Setup

- **Installation of Gutters and Downspouts:** To channel rainfall from the roof into the collection system, install gutters and downspouts. To avoid leaks and clogs, make sure the slope and alignment are correct.

- **Tank Installation:** Make sure storage tanks or cisterns are level and securely positioned when you position and install them. Excavation and construction will be needed for subterranean systems.

- **Filtration and Treatment:** Prior to storing rainwater, install filtration systems to get rid of debris and treat it. Potable water may require additional treatment, such as purification and disinfection.

- **Upkeep**

- **Regular Inspection:** To guarantee correct operation and avoid contamination, periodically clean and inspect gutters, filters, and storage tanks.

- **Keep an Eye on Water Quality:** In particular, if harvested rainwater is utilised for cooking or drinking, it is important to periodically test its purity. Deal with any contamination problems as soon as possible.

- **System Repairs**: To preserve effectiveness and water purity, fix any leaks or damage to the system's components.

5. Regulatory and Legal Aspects

- **Regulations Localised**

- **Check restrictions:** Examine building rules and municipal restrictions before installing a rainwater harvesting system. Rainwater collection systems may be subject to limitations or specifications in certain locations.

- **Permissions:** Obtain any required licenses or permissions from the relevant local authorities. Ensuring that the system is implemented and operated legally is ensured by compliance with legislation.

- **Standards for Water Quality**

- **Potable Water Standards:** Make sure the system satisfies local health and safety requirements for potable water quality if you're collecting rainwater for consumption. Additional filtering and treatment procedures could be required for this.

With a number of practical, financial, and environmental advantages, rainwater harvesting is a realistic and sustainable approach to managing water supplies. People can lessen their dependency on municipal water supplies, cut utility expenses, and promote environmental conservation by collecting and using rainwater.

In order to ensure successful and efficient operation, rainwater harvesting system implementation requires thorough planning, design, and maintenance. Rainwater collecting offers a significant chance to advance resource efficiency and sustainability, whether via subsurface systems, surface harvesting, or rooftop collection. Adopting this approach contributes to a more sustainable future and safeguards future generations' access to essential water resources.

➢ Effective Irrigation Methods: Optimising Water Utilisation for Well-Being Gardens

Effective irrigation methods are essential for maintaining healthy plant development, saving money, and conserving water. These methods reduce the amount of water wasted, make the most use of the resources at hand, and improve the sustainability of gardening and farming processes. This section examines several excellent irrigation techniques, their advantages, and useful advice for putting them into practice.

1. Gaining Knowledge About Effective Irrigation

Using techniques and tools created to maximise soil and plant health, reduce waste, and provide water to plants in the most efficient way are all part of efficient irrigation. Applying the appropriate amount of water where and when it is needed, depending on variables including soil type, plant requirements, and weather circumstances, is the main goal of efficient irrigation systems.

The advantages of effective irrigation

- **Water Conservation:** Applying water directly to the root zone and minimising evaporation and runoff reduces the amount of water used overall.

- **Cost Savings:** Minimises the need for additional irrigation and water costs.

- **Enhanced Plant Health:** Makes certain that plants have enough water to grow to their full potential, making them more resistant to illnesses and drought.

- **Environmental Impact:** Lessens the environmental impact of gardening and agriculture while also minimising the demand on nearby water supplies.

2. Different Types of Effective Irrigation Methods

1. Use of drip irrigation

- How It Works: Using a system of emitters and tubing, drip irrigation applies water straight to the roots of plants. Water is applied accurately and gently to reduce runoff and evaporation.

Advantages:
- Water Efficiency: Extremely effective at directing water to its precise location.

- Reduced Weeds: By restricting the amount of water that reaches the plant area, weed growth in unplanted regions is inhibited.

- Adaptability: Suitable for a variety of plants and garden sizes.

- Installation: Attach emitters situated close to the base of every plant to a mainline or feeder line. Maintain the system and look for clogs on a regular basis.

2. Waterproof Hoses

- **How They Operate:** Water is gradually released along the length of porous hoses via soaker hoses. To ensure even moisture distribution, they are either buried under mulch or spread out on the soil's surface.

Advantages:
- **Simplicity:** Simple to assemble and reposition as required.

- **Even Distribution:** Waters garden beds consistently.

- **Decreased Evaporation:** Water is applied in proximity to the soil's top.

- **Installation:** Arrange the hose along plant rows or in a serpentine style. Once connected to a water supply, modify the flow as necessary.

3. Sprinkler Systems

- **How They Work:** Sprinkler systems apply a fine mist or stream to a predetermined area using pressurised water. They cover a large area and can be either stationary or rotating.

Advantages:
- **Surface:** Suitable for expansive lawns and gardens.

- **Versatility:** Adaptable to various plant requirements and garden configurations.

- **Convenience:** Uses controls and timers to automate watering.

- **Installation:** Make sure the sprinklers are distributed evenly by setting them up to cover the desired area. To automate watering schedules and modify flow, use timers and controllers.

4. Watering Below the Surface

- **How It Works:** The process of subsurface irrigation entails burying tubes or water delivery lines beneath the soil. By applying water directly to the root zone, surface runoff and evaporation are decreased.

Advantages:
- **Water Efficiency:** Reduces deep percolation loss and evaporation.

- **Reduced Soil Erosion:** By delivering water below the surface, soil erosion is lessened.

- **Enhanced Root Development:** Promotes the growth of deep roots by supplying water to the root zone.

- **Installation:** Make sure to evenly space irrigation tubes or pipes by burying them beneath the soil's surface. Utilise pressure regulators and filters to keep the system operating efficiently.

3. Recommended Methods for Effective Irrigation

1. Watering Timetable

- **Timing:** To minimise evaporation losses, water in the early morning or late evening. Steer clear of watering in the heat of the day.

The frequency of watering should be adjusted according to the needs of the plants, the kind of soil, and the weather. Steer clear of overwatering, as this can cause root issues and waste water.

2. Control of Soil Moisture

- **Soil Testing:** To ascertain when to water, test the moisture content of the soil on a regular basis. To measure soil moisture, use soil probes or other basic equipment like moisture sensors.

- **Mulching:** Use mulch around plants to prevent weed growth, preserve soil moisture, and lessen evaporation. Wood chips and straw make good organic mulches.

3. Watering Methods That Work

- **Avoid Over-Spraying:** Direct hoses and sprinklers to target particular areas to prevent water waste on unplanted areas.

- **Use Gauges for Rain:** To avoid overwatering, measure the amount of water that the sprinklers apply and make adjustments to the system.

4. Upkeep of the System

- **Regular Checks:** Look for damage, obstructions, and leaks in irrigation systems. To guarantee peak performance, components should be maintained and repaired as needed.

- **Modifications:** Adjust system parameters and watering schedules in accordance with seasonal variations and plant growth phases.

4. Innovations and Technology

1. Intelligent Watering Systems

- **Features:** To optimise watering schedules and conserve water, smart irrigation systems use soil moisture sensors, programmable controllers, and weather data.

Advantages:
- **Automation:** Watering is automatically adjusted in response to current conditions.

- **Efficiency:** Minimises water waste by adapting to soil moisture levels and weather patterns.

2. Sensors of Soil Moisture

- **How They Work:** Soil moisture sensors gather information to modify irrigation schedules by measuring the moisture content of the soil.

Advantages:

- **Precision:** Enables targeted watering by giving precise information on soil moisture.

- **Water Savings:** By offering real-time data, this method lessens overwatering.

3. Sensors for Rain

- **How They Operate:** When enough rain has fallen, rain sensors sense the fall and automatically halt irrigation.

Advantages:
- **Water Conservation:** Avoids watering plants needlessly during or after precipitation.

- **Cost Savings:** Lowers utility expenses and water consumption.

Efficient irrigation techniques are critical to maximising water utilisation, improving plant health, and advancing environmentally friendly gardening and farming methods. People can save water, cut expenses, and support environmental sustainability by using techniques including subsurface irrigation, drip irrigation, soaker hoses, and sprinkler systems.

The efficiency and efficacy of irrigation operations can be further increased by using best practices, keeping up with irrigation systems, and making use of cutting-edge technologies. In light of the growing concern over water shortages and the environment, effective irrigation systems offer a workable way to manage water resources and maintain vibrant, healthy gardens and landscapes.

Chapter 3

Sustainable Materials: Creating a More Eco-Friendly Tomorrow

The expanding drive towards eco-friendly construction and design is centred around sustainable resources. These materials are selected to contribute to a more sustainable and healthy built environment while having the least possible negative effects on the environment during manufacturing and disposal. This section discusses the fundamentals of sustainable materials, looks at a variety of kinds, and offers helpful advice on how to use them in construction and design.

1. Gaining Knowledge About Sustainable Materials

Sustainable materials are those that put long-term viability, resource efficiency, and environmental responsibility first when they are utilised in manufacture, design, and building. Their capacity to mitigate adverse effects on the environment, preserve natural resources, and enhance human health and welfare is what sets them apart.

- **Most Important Sustainable Materials Concepts**

- **Resource Efficiency:** The manufacturing, processing, and transportation of sustainable materials need less resources. They frequently contain elements that are quickly renewable or recycled.

- **Low Environmental Impact:** Throughout their lifecycle, these materials produce little waste, use less energy, and emit fewer greenhouse gases than other materials.

- **Length and Durability:** Sustainable materials are made to endure a long time, which lowers the need for regular replacements and repairs.

- **Health and Safety:** By eliminating dangerous chemicals and contaminants, they help create healthier indoor environments.

2. Categories of Eco-Friendly Materials

- **Materials Recycled**

- **Definition:** Materials that have been recycled come from used goods or byproducts that have been treated and repurposed for different uses.

- ****Instances**:** Reclaimed wood, recycled steel, recycled glass, and recycled plastic.

Advantages:
- **Reduces garbage:** This lessens the requirement for virgin resources by diverting garbage from landfills.

- **Conserves Resources:** Reduces the need for energy and raw materials needed for production.

- **Decreases Environmental Impact:** Lowers the environmental impact of mining and producing materials.

- **Materials That Renew Quickly**

- **Definition:** Materials that recover rapidly within a few years are derived from plants or other biological sources.

- **Instances:** straw, cork, and bamboo.

Advantages:
- **Sustainable Growth:** These resources grow swiftly and may be extracted with little harm to ecosystems.-

- **Carbon Sequestration:** As a part of their growth, plants sequester carbon dioxide, which helps to mitigate the effects of climate change.

- **Biodegradability:** At the conclusion of their life cycle, a lot of quickly renewable materials can be recycled or biodegraded.

- **Organic and Natural Substances**

- **Definition:** Natural materials come from the soil and consist of organic molecules that are processed without undergoing chemical alteration.

- **Instances:** Wool, natural stone, clay, and wood.

Advantages:
- **Minimum Environmental Impact:** Frequently use less energy to process and include fewer artificial additives.

- **Health Benefits:** Usually devoid of dangerous chemicals and improving the quality of the air indoors.

- **Aesthetic attractiveness:** Natural materials enhance the visual attractiveness of places since they frequently have distinctive textures and colours.

- **Non-Toxic and Low-Emission Materials**

- **Definition:** These materials are made to release as few toxins or pollutants as possible into the surrounding air, especially indoors.

- **Instances:** Paints with low volatile organic compounds (VOCs), plywood without formaldehyde, and non-toxic adhesives.

Advantages:
- **Enhanced Indoor Air Quality:** Minimises exposure to dangerous substances that may have an adverse effect on health.

- **Sustainable Practices:** Encourages healthier living conditions and safer production methods.

3. Sustainable Materials' Applications

- **Construction of buildings**

- **Structural Elements:** Strong and long-lasting materials that have minimal negative effects on the environment are utilised for structural elements, such as low-impact concrete, recycled steel, and engineered wood products.

- **Insulation:** Low-impact, effective insulation can be obtained from materials like cork, sheep's wool, and cellulose, which is derived from recycled paper.

- **Finishes and Fixtures:** Reclaimed wood finishes, natural stone tiles, and low-VOC paints improve aesthetics and promote sustainability.

- **Design for the interior**

- **Furniture:** Sturdy and environmentally friendly furniture is made from natural fibres, repurposed metal, and wood that has been sourced sustainably.

- **Textiles:** Recycled polyester, bamboo, and organic cotton are common materials for curtains and upholstery since they are comfortable and have a minimal impact on the environment.

- **Flooring:** Eco-friendly and fashionable flooring materials include bamboo, cork, and reclaimed wood.

- **Garden Design**

- **Hardscaping:** Permeable paving, recycled bricks, and crushed stone are locally or recycled materials used for retaining walls, patios, and walkways.

- **Plantings**: To save water and maintain regional ecosystems, native plants and drought-tolerant species are selected.

4. Using Sustainable Resources

- **Investigation and Choosing**

- **Material Specifications:** Verify that the materials fulfil sustainability requirements by looking over environmental certificates, such as the Forest Stewardship Council (FSC) for wood or the Cradle to Cradle accreditation for items.

- **Supplier Assessment:** Select manufacturers and suppliers who have transparent supply chains and robust sustainability policies.

- **Incorporation of Design**

- **Lifecycle Assessment:** Take into account a material's complete lifecycle, from extraction and production to use and disposal. Select materials with low environmental effect and long-term benefits.

- **Strategies of Design:** Use materials in ways that will optimise their benefits; for example, choose durable finishes that require less care or use recycled content when it is structurally advantageous.

- **Knowledge and Sensitisation**

Training: Provide information on the uses and advantages of sustainable materials to architects, builders, and designers.

- **Awareness of Consumers:** Encourage the use of sustainable materials in residential and commercial projects by educating consumers about their significance.

5. Problems and Their Fixes

- **Regarding Expenses**

Difficulty: The cost of sustainable materials might occasionally exceed that of conventional alternatives.
Solution: Consider the long-term advantages, which can balance the higher initial expenditures. These advantages include lower maintenance costs and energy savings.

- **Chain of Supply and Availability**

Difficulty: Obtaining certain sustainable resources may be difficult or necessitate intricate supply systems.
Solution: Look into regional vendors and investigate substitute resources that provide comparable eco-friendly advantages.

- **Visual Appeal and Function**

Difficulty: Ensuring sustainable materials satisfy aesthetic and performance requirements.

Solution: Examine materials in a range of applications and speak with specialists to identify solutions that meet performance and design objectives.

Sustainable materials are essential to the advancement of environmentally responsible manufacturing, design, and construction techniques. Individuals and organisations may help create a greener, healthier future by selecting materials that prioritise low environmental impact, resource efficiency, and health and safety.

A wide range of sustainable options, from natural and low-emission materials to recycled and quickly regenerated resources, provide workable solutions for a number of applications. The advantages of using these materials—from financial savings to environmental preservation—make the effort worthwhile, even though it calls for careful material selection, design integration, and continual education.

Adopting sustainable materials promotes a healthy planet and sets a good example for future generations as the need for sustainability keeps rising. Through informed decision-making and promoting environmentally conscious behaviours, we can create a world that is more resilient and sustainable.

➢ Environmentally Friendly Building Materials: Opening the Door to Sustainable Building

Driven by a growing awareness of environmental effect and the need for sustainable practices, the construction industry has undergone a dramatic transition with the rise of eco-friendly building materials. These materials aim to create a healthier interior environment, minimise emissions, and use less resources. The main features of environmentally friendly building materials are examined in this part, along with their varieties, advantages, and uses.

1. Understanding Materials for Eco-Friendly Construction

Eco-friendly building materials are those that are chosen for use in construction projects on the basis of their sustainability, resource efficiency, and influence on the environment. These materials have been selected because they can help create healthy, energy-efficient buildings while minimising environmental damage during manufacturing, use, and disposal.

- **Elementary Properties of Sustainable Construction Materials**

- **Sustainability:** Made using recyclable or renewable materials and with an eye on minimising environmental impact.

- **Energy Efficiency:** Insulate buildings, use less energy, or improve thermal performance to make a positive impact on energy efficiency.

- **Low Emissions:** Reduce overall environmental impact and improve indoor air quality by emitting fewer dangerous compounds or pollutants.

- **Durability:** Provide long-lasting functionality, cutting down on waste and the need for regular replacements.

2. Eco-Friendly Construction Material Types

- **Materials that are Recycled and Reclaimed**

- **Definition:** Materials that are recycled from earlier goods or applications, cutting down on waste and the demand for fresh resources.

- **Instances:** Rubber that has been processed again, recycled steel, reclaimed wood, and recycled glass tiles.

Advantages:

- **Waste Reduction:** lessens the need for raw materials by diverting waste from landfills.

- **Resource Conservation:** Reduces the requirement for the extraction and processing of fresh materials.

- **Unique Aesthetics:** These give designs individuality and frequently possess unique traits and historical significance.

- **2. Materials That Renew Quickly**

- **Definition:** Materials derived from rapidly growing plants or other renewable resources that can be gathered in a brief amount of time.

- **Instances :** straw bales, cork, and bamboo.

Advantages:
- **Quick Regrowth:** May be restored rapidly, lessening the burden on ecosystems.

- **Carbon Sequestration:** As a result of their growth, plants sequester carbon dioxide, which slows down global warming.

- **Biodegradability:** Recyclable or biodegradable materials are abundant in quickly renewable resources.

- **Organic and Natural Substances**

- **Definition:** Natural materials are those that come from the source with little to no processing or chemical additions.

- **Examples:** Wool, wood, clay, and natural stone.

Advantages:
- **Low Environmental Impact:** They don't contain artificial chemicals and often require less energy to process.

- **Healthier Indoor Air Quality:** Toxins and volatile organic compounds (VOCs) are typically absent from natural materials.

- **Aesthetic Appeal:** Enhance the visual appeal of areas with distinctive textures and natural beauty.

- **Non-Toxic and Low-Emission Materials**

- **Definition:** Materials made to release the fewest amount of harmful compounds or pollutants possible, enhancing indoor air quality and environmental safety.

- **Examples:** Non-toxic adhesives, plywood free of formaldehyde, and low-VOC paints.

Advantages:

- **Improved Indoor Air Quality:** Lowers exposure to dangerous substances and impurities.

- **Health Benefits:** Lowers the risk of respiratory problems and promotes healthier living conditions.

- **Materials for Insulation**

- **Definition:** Components that improve the energy efficiency and thermal performance of a building.

- **Examples:** cork, sheep's wool, and cellulose (produced from recycled paper).

Advantages:
- **Energy Savings:** Enhances thermal insulation to lower heating and cooling expenses.

- **Sustainability:** Frequently produced using resources that are quickly renewable or recycled.

- **Soundproofing:** Offers acoustic advantages to improve seclusion and comfort.

3. Utilising Eco-Friendly Construction Materials

- **Building for Residential Use**

- **Exterior Finishes:** Using environmentally friendly siding materials, including fiber-cement siding, salvaged wood, or natural stone, improves appearance and longevity while reducing impact on the environment.

- **Interior Finishes:** Eco-friendly materials help create elegant interior designs and healthier indoor environments. Examples include low-VOC paints, bamboo flooring, and recycled glass tiles.

- **Insulation:** To increase energy efficiency and save utility costs, use sustainable insulation materials.

- 2. **Building for Commercial Use**

- **Structural Elements:** Utilising green concrete, engineered wood products, and recycled steel for structural elements helps achieve sustainability objectives while improving building performance.

- **Facades and Roofing:** To reduce energy consumption and minimise environmental effect, employ sustainable materials for building facades and green roofing solutions, such as cool or living roofs.

- **Décoration within:** To create a healthier and more sustainable workspace, choose environmentally friendly materials for office furnishings, partitions, and finishes.

- **Outdoor Spaces and Landscaping**

- **Hardscaping:** For patios, pathways, and retaining walls, choose eco-friendly materials such as permeable pavers, recycled aggregate, and reclaimed bricks.

- **Plantings:** To save water and promote regional ecosystems, select native and drought-tolerant plants.

- **Water Features:** To improve outdoor areas while preserving resources, use recycled water systems and environmentally friendly materials for fountains and ponds.

4. Using Sustainable Construction Materials**

- **Selection of Materials**

- **Research:** Look into the sustainability ratings and environmental certifications of materials, such as LEED (Leadership in Energy and Environmental Design) and Cradle to Cradle.

- **Local Sourcing:** To lower emissions associated with transportation and boost local economies, choose materials that are supplied locally.

- **Supplier Evaluation:** Select vendors who have transparent supply chains and robust environmental policies.

- **Incorporation of Design**

- **Lifecycle Assessment:** Take into account the full lifecycle of materials, from extraction and manufacture to disposal, and select solutions that have the least negative effects on the environment.

- **Strategies of Design:** Use sustainable materials in methods that improve functionality and appearance, such as selecting durable finishes to lower maintenance requirements or employing recycled content where it adds value.

- **Knowledge and Sensitisation**

- **Training:** Inform designers, architects, and builders on the uses and advantages of environmentally friendly materials.

- **Awareness of Consumers:** Encourage the use of eco-friendly materials in residential and commercial projects and educate consumers about the value of sustainable building methods.

5. Problems and Their Fixes

- **Regarding Expenses**

- **Challenge:** Compared to traditional solutions, eco-friendly materials might occasionally be more expensive up front.

- **Remedy:** Consider the long-term advantages that can outweigh the initial expenses, such as lower maintenance requirements, improved health, and energy savings.

- **Chain of Supply and Availability**

- **Difficulty:** A few environmentally friendly items might not be readily available or have convoluted supply networks.

- **Remedy:** Look into regional vendors and investigate substitute materials that provide comparable eco-friendly advantages.

- **Visual Appeal and Function**

- **Difficulty:** Ensuring that environmentally friendly materials live up to performance and aesthetic standards.

- **Solution:** Examine materials in a range of applications and speak with specialists to identify solutions that meet performance and design objectives.

Buildings that are resource-efficient, healthful, and sustainable must be made with eco-friendly materials. Building more sustainable communities and making a positive influence on the environment are possible for individuals and organisations that choose materials that prioritise indoor air quality, resource conservation, and environmental impact.

The array of environmentally friendly options provides workable solutions for a range of building and design needs, from recycled and quickly renewable resources to natural and low-emission materials. Although putting these materials into practice involves careful selection, design integration, and continuing education, the rewards—which include better health, lower environmental impact, and financial savings—make the effort worthwhile.

Adopting eco-friendly materials is a positive example for future generations and supports sustainability goals as the building industry continues to change. We can design structures that are not only attractive and useful, but also in line with the values of sustainability and environmental care by educating ourselves and pushing for greener methods.

➢ Low-VOC Paints: Improving Sustainability and Indoor Air Quality

A big step forward in the direction of greener, more sustainable building techniques is low-VOC paint. Volatile organic compounds, or VOCs, are substances that some solids or liquids, including conventional paints, can release as gases. These emissions may be harmful to one's health and lead to indoor air pollution. Paints labelled as low-VOC are made to reduce these emissions, providing a greener and safer substitute. The qualities, advantages, uses, and considerations of low-VOC paints are examined in this section.

1. Comprehending the Effects of VOCs

A class of organic compounds known as volatile organic compounds (VOCs) evaporate readily at ambient temperature. VOCs are employed as solvents in paints and varnishes to dissolve other chemicals and make application easier. VOCs are released into the air when paint dries, and this can lead to air pollution both indoors and outdoors.

- **Environmental and Health Risks**

- **Health impacts:** VOC exposure can result in a variety of health concerns, such as headaches, dizziness, respiratory disorders, and in certain situations, long-term health impacts like kidney and liver damage. Additionally, some VOCs are known or suspected carcinogens.

- **Environmental Impact:** VOCs are involved in the creation of ground-level ozone, a major cause of smog that can be detrimental to the environment and human health.

2. Low-VOC Paint Features

- **Explanation and Guidelines**

- **Low-VOC Paints:** Compared to conventional paints, these paints have fewer volatile organic chemicals in their formulation. Low-VOC paints normally have between 50 and 250 grams of volatile organic compounds (VOCs) per litre, depending on the type and application. The precise VOC content is regulated and varies by location.

- **Standards and Certifications:** Low-VOC and zero-VOC paints are certified by a number of agencies and initiatives, including Green Seal and the Environmental Protection Agency (EPA).

Principal Features

- **Reduced Emissions:** Lower volatile organic compounds (VOCs) released by low-VOC paints improve indoor air quality.

- **Quick Drying:** Low-VOC paints can be used in both residential and commercial environments since they often dry faster than conventional paints.

- **Performance and Durability:** Thanks to developments in paint science, low-VOC paints are now as durable, opaque, and aesthetically pleasing as conventional paints.

3. Low-VOC Paints' Advantages

- Health Advantages

- **Improved Indoor Air Quality:** These paints contribute to a better living environment by lowering the concentration of dangerous pollutants in indoor air by releasing less volatile organic compounds.

- **Reduced Allergens and Irritants:** Low-VOC paints are a better option for sensitive people, such as children and those with underlying medical conditions, because they are less likely to result in respiratory problems or allergic responses.

- **Advantages for the Environment**

- **Lower Contribution to Smog:** Lowering VOC emissions improves outdoor air quality by preventing the production of smog and ground-level ozone.

- **Sustainability:** A lot of low-VOC paints are produced using sustainable methods and eco-friendly materials, which lessens their overall impact on the environment.

- **Practical and Aesthetic Advantages**

- **Wide Range of Options:** Low-VOC paints provide you versatility in design and application because they are available in a variety of colours, finishes, and types.

- **Ease of Use:** Thanks to advancements in paint technology, low-VOC paints are just as durable, easy to apply, and provide good coverage as traditional paints.

4. Low-VOC Paint Applications

- Interiors of Residential Buildings

- **Living Spaces:** Low-VOC paints work well in living spaces—like bedrooms, living rooms, and kitchens—where people spend a lot of time in the house.

- **Children's Rooms:** Low-VOC paints are a better option for painting nurseries and kids' rooms due to their lower health concerns.

- Institutional and Commercial Buildings

- **Offices and Schools:** To create healthier work and learning environments, low-VOC paints are being employed in commercial and institutional buildings more and more.

- **Healthcare Facilities:** Low-VOC paints improve indoor air quality and promote patient health in hospitals and clinics.

- **Remodelling and Renovation**

- **Restoration Projects:** Low-VOC paints can help lessen the negative effects of renovations on the environment and human health in older buildings.

- **Green Building Certifications:** LEED (Leadership in Energy and Environmental Design) and other green building standards and certifications can be attained with the use of low-VOC paints.

5. Selection and Application of Low-VOC Paints

- **Selection Standards**

- **Check VOC Levels:** Make sure the paint satisfies low-VOC requirements by checking its VOC content.

- **Check Certifications and Labels:** To learn about the health and environmental benefits of paint, study product labels and look for certifications from reliable organisations.

- **Compare Results:** To make sure the paint fits the requirements of your project, consider aspects like durability, drying time, and coverage.

- **Application Hints**

- **Ventilation:** To maintain high air quality, even if low-VOC paints are less toxic, it's still vital to make sure there is enough ventilation both before and after application.

- **Surface Setting Up:** To guarantee excellent adhesion and durability and to get the best effects, surfaces should be painted with care.

- **Care:** To extend the life and appearance of the paint, adhere to the cleaning and care guidelines provided by the manufacturer.

- **Examining Expenses**

- **Price Comparison:** Although the cost of low-VOC paints can occasionally exceed that of conventional alternatives, the advantages in terms of health and environmental impact frequently outweigh the price.

- **Long-Term benefits:** Take into account the financial benefits over time that come with lower health risks and better indoor air quality.

6. Problems and Their Fixes

- Price

- **Difficulty:** The cost of low-VOC paints can be higher than that of conventional paints.

- **Solution:** Compare brands to identify affordable solutions and assess the total value, taking into account potential long-term savings and health benefits.

- **Restricted Stock**

- **Difficulty:** Not every paint retailer may have an extensive assortment of low-VOC paints.

- **Solution:** Look into online resources and providers to locate a range of low-VOC paints that satisfy your requirements.

- **Issues with Performance**

- **Challenge:** Concerns over low-VOC paints' performance in comparison to conventional choices may exist among certain customers.

- **Remedy:** To make sure the paint fulfils performance requirements, test samples, read reviews, and get advice from experts.

Low-VOC paints, which provide a healthier substitute for conventional paints, mark a substantial improvement in sustainable building methods. These paints are essential for creating safer, more environmentally friendly living and working environments because they lower harmful emissions, enhance indoor air quality, and support environmental sustainability.

Choosing and using low-VOC paints requires knowledge of their advantages, product selection, and efficient application. Notwithstanding these difficulties, low-VOC paints are a wise investment for both residential and commercial projects because of their many benefits, which include better health, less of an adverse effect on the environment, and possible cost savings.

Low-VOC paints will continue to be essential to attaining these objectives as the demand for greener and healthier building methods grows. Individuals and organisations may promote healthier interior conditions for everyone and contribute to a more sustainable future by adopting these environmentally friendly solutions.

➢ Eco-Friendly Living Spaces: Furnishings and Décor Made of Sustainable Materials

The trend towards sustainability is still influencing many areas of our lives, and interior design and furnishings are no exception. Sustainable furnishings and décor prioritise reducing their negative effects on the environment, supporting moral behaviour, and improving occupant well-being. The fundamentals of sustainable furniture and décor are covered in this area, along with important materials, design considerations, and useful advice for furnishing eco-friendly homes.

1. Comprehending Eco-Friendly Furniture and Design

Sustainable furnishings and décor are created with an emphasis on lessening their negative effects on the environment and promoting moral behaviour. This entails minimising waste, employing environmentally friendly materials, and making sure that fair labour standards are met during product manufacturing. The objective is to design living areas that are in line with sustainability and responsibility ideals in addition to being fashionable and practical.

- **Principles Essential to Sustainability**

- **Resource Efficiency:** Make use of supplies and procedures that reduce waste and resource use.

- **Durability:** Select items that are sturdy and less likely to require replacements over time.

- **Recyclability and Reusability:** Choose products that, at the end of their useful lives, may be recycled or put to new uses.

- **Production Ethics:** Make sure that the production of furniture and décor has a minimal impact on the environment and adheres to fair labour practices.

2. Sustainable Furniture Materials

- **Materials that are Recycled and Reclaimed**

Definition: Materials that are recycled from earlier goods or applications, cutting down on waste and the demand for fresh resources.
Repurposed fabrics, recycled metal, and reclaimed wood are a few examples.

Advantages:
Waste Reduction: lessens the need for virgin resources by diverting materials from landfills.

Singular Personality: Reclaimed materials provide designs character because they frequently have distinct aesthetics and historical significance.

- **Resources that are Renewable and Quickly Renewable**

Definition: Materials that come from naturally renewable sources or sources that can be swiftly renewed.

Instances: Wool, cork, and bamboo.

Advantages:

Quick Regrowth: Materials with quick growth, such as bamboo, ease the burden on ecosystems and guarantee a steady supply.

Low Environmental Impact: Their industrial procedures frequently use less energy and fewer chemicals.

- **Low-Emission and Non-Toxic Materials**

Definition: Substances that enhance indoor air quality by being devoid of dangerous chemicals and contaminants.

Examples: Organic cotton, natural latex, and low-VOC coatings.

Advantages:

Healthier Indoor Environment: Lowers exposure to other pollutants and volatile organic compounds (VOCs).

Improved Air Quality: Reduces the emission of hazardous pollutants, making living spaces healthier.

- **Materials Repurposed**

Definition: Materials that are inventively recycled from trash or abandoned objects to make brand-new, useful things.

Examples: Reclaimed glass transformed into ornamental pieces, and upcycled furniture constructed from used pallets.

Advantages:

Creative and Unique: Provides chances for personalised and unique designs.

Reduction of Waste: Gives discarded goods a new use, which helps cut down on the quantity of garbage dumped in landfills.

3. Considering Sustainability While Designing

- **Classic Style**

Concept: Emphasise timeless, classic styles that will not rapidly go out of style.

Advantages:

Longevity: Makes furniture and décor last longer by lowering the need for regular upgrades and replacements.

Versatility: Classical works are easily adaptable to a variety of situations and styles.

- **Multipurpose and Modular Furniture**

Concept: Select furniture with numerous uses or that is easily reconfigurable.

Advantages:
Adaptability: Minimises the need for extra pieces and permits flexible living arrangements.

Space Efficiency: Perfect for apartments and smaller houses with constrained space.

- **Handcrafted and Regional Goods**

Concept: Buy locally produced goods to show your support for regional manufacturers and artists.

Advantages:
Reduced Transport Emissions: lessens the shipping industry's carbon footprint.

Economic Support: Encourages traditional craft skills and strengthens local economies.

- **Green Production Techniques**

Concept: Choose goods from manufacturers who value ethical and sustainable production methods.

Advantages:

Lower Environmental Impact: Environmental footprints of manufacturers who employ eco-friendly practices are frequently smaller overall.

Ethical Standards: Guarantees ethical labour methods and conscientious material sourcing.

4. Useful Advice for Eco-Friendly Furniture and Décor

- **Make Quality Your Top Priority**

Advise: Make a wise investment in long-lasting, well-made items.

Advantages:

Long-Term Savings: Minimises the frequency of repairs and replacements.

Environmental Impact: Reductions in waste and resource usage result from fewer replacements.

- Look for Vintage and Used Items

Tip: Look for distinctive, previously owned objects in antique stores, thrift stores, and online markets.

Advantages:

Preservation of Resources: reuses current items and lowers the need for new production.

Unique Finds: Provides a large selection of eye-catching, frequently reasonably priced items.

- **Handmade and Repurposed Items**

Tip: Use your imagination when working on do-it-yourself projects and upcycling materials to create fresh décor out of old furniture.

Advantages:

Customisation: Enables unique touches and custom designs.

Trash Reduction: Recycles old items and cuts down on trash.

- **Select Fabrics and Finishes with Minimal Impact**

Tip: Choose textiles and finishes made of natural or recycled materials that have minimal volatile organic compounds (VOCs).

Advantages:

Health Advantages: lowers chemical emissions to improve indoor air quality.

Impact on the Environment: reduces the usage of dangerous chemicals and encourages environmentally friendly behaviour.

- **5. Encourage Brands to Adopt Sustainable Practices**

Tip: Look up and select brands who put sustainability first in their sourcing, manufacturing, and commercial procedures.

Advantages:
Ethical Consumption: Make sure your purchases are in line with moral and environmental principles.

Encouraging Best Practices: Provides assistance to businesses setting the standard for sustainability.

5. Problems and Their Fixes

- **Regarding Expenses**

Challenge: Compared to conventional solutions, sustainable furniture and design might occasionally cost more.

Remedy: Think about the long-term advantages of longevity and less environmental effect, and look into used options for more cost-effective possibilities.

- **Restricted Stock**

Difficulty: Not every merchant may have a large assortment of eco-friendly goods.

Solution: Look into specialty shops and internet merchants that provide ethical and environmentally friendly goods.

- **Ethical Issues**

Challenge: Conventional design choices might not be compatible with all sustainable materials.

Solution: Adopt contemporary design styles that use eco-friendly materials, and investigate creative concepts that draw attention to the special features of environmentally friendly goods.

Designing eco-friendly and fashionable living spaces with sustainable furniture and decor is a powerful approach to uphold moral and ethical standards. People may make a difference in a more sustainable future by adopting design principles that reduce waste and boost local economies, as well as by selecting materials that prioritise durability, non-toxicity, and resource efficiency.

Putting into practice sustainable furniture and décor calls for careful planning, innovative design, and a dedication to long-term worth. The advantages of sustainable options, which range from better indoor air quality to less environmental effect, outweigh the drawbacks, such as cost and availability.

There will probably be even more innovations and possibilities in the furniture and design sector as the demand for eco-friendly items grows, which will make it simpler for customers to make sustainable decisions. By adopting these techniques, we may create living environments that are in line with our ethical and environmental beliefs in addition to being aesthetically pleasing and practical.

Chapter 4

Waste Reduction: Techniques for a Future That Is More Sustainable

A key component of environmental sustainability is waste reduction, which aims to reduce waste production and improve resource management. It entails handling, reusing, and recycling resources better in addition to cutting down on the amount of waste we produce. This section examines practical actions that people and organisations may take to decrease waste and encourage a more sustainable future, as well as successful waste reduction programs and their advantages.

1. Contemplating Reduction of Waste

- **Definition of Waste Reduction**

The term "waste reduction" describes methods and approaches intended to lower the amount of garbage produced. Instead of just handling or getting rid of garbage after it has been produced, it focusses on stopping waste from being formed in the first place. Reducing waste's negative effects on the environment, preserving resources, and advancing a circular economy—one in which products are recycled and reused—are the objectives.

- **Fundamental Ideas for Reducing Waste**

- **Source Reduction:** Make adjustments to the processes of production and consumption to stop the creation of waste.

- **Reuse:** Repair, repurpose, or direct reuse can prolong the life of materials and products.

- **Recycling:** Reduce the need for virgin resources and landfill usage by repurposing discarded materials into new goods.

- **Composting:** Convert organic waste into nutrient-rich compost to improve soil quality and promote environmentally friendly farming practices.

2. Waste Reduction Strategies

- **Diminish**

- **Reduce Consumption:** Select sturdy, long-lasting products and those with little to no packaging. Cutting back on consumption overall aids in lowering the amount of garbage generated.

- **Efficient Resource Use:** Adopt resource-saving techniques, such using energy-efficient appliances and digital documents instead of paper.

- **Wise Purchasing:** Refrain from making impulsive purchases and only buy what is required. Making grocery lists and meal plans might help cut down on food wastage.

- **Reutilise**

- **Repurpose goods:** Give discarded goods new life. For instance, old furniture can be restored or repurposed, and glass jars can be utilised as storage.

- **Secondhand Purchases:** Invest in used products including electronics, furniture, and clothes. By doing this, waste is decreased and the circular economy is strengthened.

- **Repair:** Mend damaged objects rather than throwing them away. Clothes, appliances, and gadgets can all have their lifespans greatly increased by repairs.

- **Reutilise**

- **Separate and Sort:** Sort recyclables from non-recyclables to implement efficient recycling procedures. Inform everyone, including yourself, about what can and cannot be recycled in your community.

- **Take Part in Programs:** Take part in neighbourhood recycling initiatives and drop-off locations for dangerous goods, electronics, and batteries.

- **Adopt Recycled Items:** To complete the recycling cycle and promote the markets for recycled goods, choose products manufactured from recycled resources.

- **Reusing and Recycling**

- **Organic Waste Management:** To cut down on landfill waste, compost yard debris, food scraps and other organic wastes. These materials are composted to create valuable compost that can enhance soil health.

- **Composting at Home:** Install a system at home to compost garden and kitchen trash. utilising compost bins or vermicomposting—a process that involves utilising worms—are efficient ways to handle organic waste.

- **Community Programs:** To handle organic waste on a bigger scale, take part in or encourage community composting projects.

3. Advantages of Reducing Waste

- **Advantages for the Environment**

- **Reduced Landfill Use:** Reducing the amount of waste dumped in landfills contributes to lessening greenhouse gas emissions and environmental degradation.

- **Resource Conservation:** Reducing energy use, environmental damage, and the exploitation of natural resources are all made possible by efficient resource use and recycling.

- **Pollution Reduction:** By producing less trash, hazardous materials and pollutants that could leak into the environment or be released into the air are reduced.

- **Financial Gains**

- **Cost Savings:** For both people and companies, cutting waste can result in significant cost savings. For instance, cutting back on purchases and improving trash management can save disposal expenses and increase product longevity.

- **Increased Efficiency:** Organisations that use waste reduction techniques frequently see increases in material cost savings and operational effectiveness.

- **Market Opportunities:** The need for sustainable goods and recyclable materials fosters the growth of green businesses by generating job opportunities.

- Advantages for Society

- **Enhanced Community Well-Being:** By cutting pollutants and keeping public areas cleaner, efficient waste management techniques promote healthier and cleaner communities.

- **Educational Opportunities:** Waste reduction programs offer chances for awareness-raising and education, which motivates people and businesses to embrace sustainable practices and make wise decisions.

4. Putting Waste Reduction Plans Into Practice

- **Personal Initiatives**

- **Adopt Sustainable Practices:** Make waste reduction techniques a part of your everyday routine by choosing eco-friendly products, using reusable bags, and using refillable water bottles.

- **Educate and Advocate:** Spread the word about waste reduction in the workplace, schools, and your community. Disseminate information and inspire people to embrace sustainable practices.

- **Observe and Assess:** Evaluate your waste reduction initiatives on a regular basis to find areas for improvement and monitor your success.

- **Organisational and Business Actions**

- **Create Waste Reduction Policies:** Put into action procedures and policies that give priority to reducing waste, such as sustainable procurement, resource efficiency, and zero-waste programs.

- **Involve Employees:** Encourage staff members to embrace sustainable practices and take part in recycling initiatives by educating and including them in trash reduction initiatives.

- **Assess and Document:** Monitor the production and reduction of trash, and update stakeholders on your progress. Analyse data to pinpoint areas in need of development and recognise achievements.

- **Government and Community Actions**

- **Support Programs and efforts:** Take part in and lend your support to regional waste management campaigns, recycling campaigns, and composting efforts.

- **Support Policy Changes:** Encourage laws and rules that lessen waste, such as those pertaining to extended producer responsibility (EPR) and the prohibition of single-use plastics.

- **Promote Collaboration:** Develop and implement efficient waste reduction methods in partnership with enterprises, government agencies, and community organisations.

5. Problems and Their Fixes

- **Modification of Behaviour**

- **Challenge:** Changing behaviour and habits significantly may be necessary to adopt waste reduction measures.

- **Remedy:** Encourage people and organisations to adopt waste reduction by offering incentives and education. Emphasise the advantages and provide workable solutions to make adoption easier.

- **Limitations in Infrastructure**

- **Challenge:** The efficiency of trash reduction initiatives may be hampered by inadequate infrastructure for composting and recycling.

- **Solution:** Promote better waste management infrastructure and lend assistance to neighbourhood projects that overcome these drawbacks.

- **Financial Limitations**

- **Challenge:** For some people and companies, the upfront expenses of putting waste reduction initiatives into practice can be a barrier.

- **Remedy:** Stress the advantages and long-term cost reductions of waste reduction. Approach government agencies and environmental groups for funds or assistance.

With so many advantages for the economy, society, and environment, waste reduction is an essential part of environmental sustainability. Through the implementation of tactics like consumption reduction, item reuse, material recycling, and organic waste composting, both individuals and organisations can considerably reduce their ecological footprint and foster a more sustainable future.

Putting waste reduction strategies into effect requires a mix of community, corporate, and individual efforts. The long-term advantages of trash reduction, which include resource conservation, financial savings, and enhanced community well-being, outweigh any difficulties.

The objective of a zero-waste society will continue to be advanced by creative solutions and encouraging legislation as awareness and dedication to waste reduction increase. Through adopting these habits and motivating others to follow suit, we can all contribute to the creation of a more sustainable, greener, and cleaner planet.

➢ Composting at Home: Using Waste to Create Priceless Resources

Composting at home is a sustainable method that turns organic waste into nutrient-rich compost that can improve soil quality and encourage strong plant development. People can lessen the amount of garbage they produce at home, lessen the impact landfills have on the environment, and provide a useful resource for gardening and landscaping by starting a compost at home. This manual covers the fundamentals of home composting, its advantages, and doable procedures for setting up and running a productive composting system.

1. Comprehending Composting at Home

Composting at home is the process of using natural decomposition to turn organic waste, like food scraps and yard trash, into compost. In order to transform organic material into humus—a black, nutrient-rich material that can be used to enhance soil fertility and structure—microorganisms, bacteria, fungi, and other decomposers are involved in this process.

- **Important Composting Components**

- **Organic Materials:** Food scraps, yard debris, and other biodegradable materials that break down to form compost.

- **Microorganisms:** These are the bacteria, fungi, and other microbes that aid in the composting process by decomposing organic materials.

- **Oxygen:** Aerobic decomposition, which generates compost effectively and lessens odours, requires air.

- **Moisture:** Sufficient moisture promotes the growth of microorganisms and quickens the breakdown process.

2. Advantages of Composting at Home

- **Reducing Waste**

- **Less Landfill Waste:** By composting organic waste, less material is dumped in landfills, which lowers greenhouse gas emissions and landfill overflow.

- **Resource Efficiency:** Composting allows you to make efficient use of and keep priceless organic materials out of the trash stream.

- **Enhancement of Soil**

- **Nutrient-Rich Compost:** Compost enriches the soil with vital nutrients, enhancing its fertility and structure and promoting strong plant development.

- **Improved Soil Health:** Compost assists plant roots and fosters a healthy ecosystem by enhancing soil texture, moisture retention, and aeration.

- **Advantages for the Environment**

- **Reduced Greenhouse Gas Emissions:** One of the main greenhouse gases that contributes to climate change is methane, which composting lowers emissions from landfills.

- **Resource Conservation:** By eliminating the need for chemical soil amendments and synthetic fertilisers, composting helps to preserve natural resources and lower pollution levels in the environment.

- **Financial Reductions**

- **Lower Waste Disposal Costs:** Waste management expenses may be decreased by lowering the amount of waste that is transported to disposal sites.

- **Decreased Requirement for Store-Bought Fertilisers:** Composting offers a free natural fertiliser source, negating the need to buy manufactured goods.

3. How to Begin Composting at Home

- **Selecting a Composting Technique**

Composting at home can be done in a number of ways, depending on your needs and available space:

- **Compost Bins:** Covered bins made specifically for composting. They aid in material containment, odour control, and decomposition acceleration. Tumblers, regular bins, and stackable bins are available options.

- **Compost Piles:** Composterable materials piled in an open manner. This approach is easy to use and reasonably priced, but it needs more room and ongoing supervision.

- **Vermicomposting:** This method breaks down organic waste by using worms, usually red wigglers. This method yields high-quality compost quickly and is appropriate for smaller settings.

- **Bokashi Composting:** A fermentation-based technique that breaks down organic waste in a sealed container with the help of helpful bacteria. It can handle a larger variety of materials and is appropriate for indoor composting.

- **Materials Selection for Composting**

Green Materials: Materials with a high nitrogen content that give microorganisms vital nutrition. Grass clippings, coffee grounds, and leftover fruits and vegetables are a few examples.

Brown Materials: High-carbon components that provide the compost shape and balance. Straw, cardboard, and dried leaves are a few examples.

Avoid Composting: Steer clear of things like meat, dairy, greasy foods, and pet waste that might cause issues. These may harbour infections, produce odours, and draw pests.

4. Establishing Appropriate Environments

- **Arrangement in Layers**

- **Balance Materials:** To keep the carbon-to-nitrogen ratio balanced, alternate layers of green and brown materials. Utilising around two parts brown materials to one part green materials is a typical guideline.

- **Size and Shredding:** To promote even mixing and hasten decomposition, chop or shred larger items.

- **Ventilation**

- **Turning:** To provide oxygen and hasten decomposition, stir or mix the compost on a regular basis. To mix the contents in compost bins, use a pitchfork or compost turner.

- **Ventilation:** To avoid anaerobic conditions and lessen odours, make sure there is adequate airflow by keeping the structure open or by utilising aeration tools.

- **Adequate Humidity**

- **Maintain Moisture Levels:** Don't let the compost dry up completely; instead, keep it damp. While little moisture might hinder decomposition, excessive moisture can cause sogginess and odour.

- **Modifying Moisture:** If the compost is excessively moist, add dry brown materials; if it is too dry, add water.

5. Handling the Process of Composting

- Observation

- **Temperature:** For active decomposition, compost should be heated to 130–160°F (54–71°C). This aids in eliminating weed seeds and infections.

- **Odour:** A well-kept compost pile should smell earthy and pleasant. Bad smells might be a sign of problems like too much moisture or not enough airflow.

- Diagnostics

- **Slow Decomposition:** Check moisture levels, change the material balance, or boost aeration if composting is going slowly.

- **Pests and Rodents:** Steer clear of adding meat, dairy, or fatty foods to ward off pests. Make sure the compost pile or container is contained and maintained appropriately.

- **Composter Harvesting**

- **Completion:** When the compost is crumbly, black, and smells earthy, it is ready. The original components must be unrecognisable.

- **Screening:** You might choose to filter the compost or remove any big, undecomposed objects. You can put these back into the composting system to break them down even more.

6. Making Use of Compost

- **Use in the Garden**

- **Soil Amendment:** To enhance the structure, fertility, and moisture retention of garden soil, incorporate compost into it. This promotes robust root systems and increases plant development.

- **Mulching:** To keep plants weed-free, preserve moisture, and supply nutrients, mulch them with compost.

- **Indoor Botany**

- **Potting Mix:** For indoor plants, incorporate compost into the potting mix. It gives the soil vital nutrients and enhances drainage and aeration.

- **Garden Design**

- **Erosion Control:** In landscaping projects, use compost to stabilise the soil and lessen erosion.

- **Lawn Improvement:** To enhance soil health and encourage lush, green growth, apply compost to lawns.

Composting at home is an excellent and useful method to improve soil, cut down on waste, and encourage a more sustainable way of living. Through comprehension of the fundamentals of composting, selection of an appropriate technique, and adherence to recommended standards, people can efficiently handle organic waste and provide an invaluable resource for horticulture and landscaping.

Beyond only decreasing trash, home composting has several advantages such as better soil health, environmental preservation, and financial savings. Composting can be used into a larger waste reduction plan to help create a cleaner, more sustainable future. Whether you're new to composting or want to upgrade your current setup, implementing these habits can have a big beneficial influence on both the environment and your house.

➢ Recycling & Upcycling: Creating Value Out of Waste

Reducing waste and preserving resources are the two main goals of recycling and upcycling, which are integral parts of sustainable living. Although they both aim to reduce their negative effects on the environment, their methods and results vary. This section examines the fundamentals of upcycling and recycling, as well as the advantages and doable actions involved in putting these ideas into practice.

1. Getting to Know Upcycling and Recycling

- **Reuse**

In order to make new items, recycled materials must be gathered, sorted, and processed. This procedure saves energy, lessens the demand for raw materials, and keeps garbage out of landfills. Materials including paper, glass, plastics, and metals are frequently recycled. Recycling involves disassembling these materials into their most basic parts and then reassembling them to create new goods.

- **Upcycling**

Upcycling, sometimes referred to as creative reuse, is the process of turning discarded or used materials into brand-new, more valuable goods. In contrast to recycling, which frequently necessitates industrial processing, upcycling makes use of artistry and creativity to prolong the life of materials and things. The idea is to give the original item a new function or purpose in order to increase its value.

2. Recycling and Upcycling's Advantages

- **Advantages for the Environment**

- **Resource Conservation:** Recycling helps to preserve natural resources like wood, water, and minerals by lowering the need for virgin materials. Similar to this, upcycling uses pre-existing resources to avoid the need for new ones.

- **Energy Savings:** Compared to making new items from raw materials, recycling usually uses less energy. Because upcycling eliminates the need for new item creation, it also conserves energy.

- **Trash Reduction:** Recycling and upcycling contribute to the reduction of trash delivered to incinerators and landfills, which lowers greenhouse gas emissions and pollutants.

- **Financial Gains**

- **Cost Savings:** Recycling keeps items out of landfills, which lowers waste management expenses. Because upcycling entails reusing pre-existing things, it frequently requires little financial commitment.

- **Job Creation:** The upcycling and recycling sectors generate employment in processing, creative design, sorting, and collection. This encourages sustainable business practices and supports regional economies.

- **Advantages for Society**

- **Community Engagement**: Recycling campaigns and upcycling projects encourage participation in the community and increase knowledge of environmental problems. They urge people to support regional artists and engage in sustainable behaviours.

- **Educational Opportunities:** Recycling and upcycling are two excellent ways to teach students about creativity, resource conservation, and environmental care.

3. **Recycling Procedures and Recommended Approaches**

- **The Reclamation Procedure**

- **Collection:** Recycling bins, drop-off locations, and curbside pickup are the methods used to gather recyclables.

- **Sorting:** To guarantee appropriate processing, materials are classified into categories (such as paper, glass, and plastic). To make recycled materials of higher grade, contaminants are eliminated.

- **Processing:** Materials that have been sorted are converted into raw materials so that new products can be made. This could entail melting, shredding, or other techniques.

- **Manufacturing:** By utilising recycled raw materials to make new goods, the recycling cycle is completed and less fresh material is required.

- **Recycle with Best Practices**

- **Know What Can Be Recycled:** Make sure the things you want to recycle are accepted by your community's recycling program by familiarising yourself with its recycling policies.

- **Correct Arrangement:** Sort recyclables from non-recyclables and get rid of anything that can impede recycling, like plastic bags and food residue.

- **Minimise Pollution:** To increase the effectiveness and quality of recycling, rinse out containers and refrain from combining different kinds of recyclables.

- **Materials Often Recycled**

- **Paper:** Consists of office paper, cardboard, periodicals, and newspapers. Paper that has been recycled can be used to make new paper goods or packaging materials.

- **Glass:** Glass jars and bottles that are clear, green, or brown can be recycled to make new glassware.

- **Plastics:** Bottles, containers, and packaging are examples of common plastics. Plastics are recyclable and can be made into new materials or products based on the type of resin they contain.

- **Metals:** Steel and aluminium cans are precious recyclable materials that can be refined to create new metal goods.

4. Upcycling: Innovative and Creative Reuse

- **Ideas for Upcycling**

- **Furniture and Home Decor:** Sand, paint, or reupholster old furniture to give it new life. Repurpose waste materials like wooden pallets and old suitcases to create chic storage solutions or home décor.

- **Apparel and Accessory:** Repurpose outdated garments to create chic things, like transforming t-shirts into tote bags or jeans into skirts. Refresh worn items with imaginative changes or additions.

- **Craft Projects:** Make handcrafted gifts, crafts, or artwork out of leftover fabric, bottle caps, and paper rolls. Upcycling promotes creativity and makes unique, customised items possible.

- **Advantages of Repurposing**

- **Waste Reduction:** By giving objects a new lease of life and extending their useful life, upcycling keeps them out of landfills.

- **Unique Products:** Repurposed goods frequently stand out from mass-produced things due to their distinctive, handcrafted nature. This gives commonplace objects more aesthetic and utilitarian value.

- **Cost-Effective:** For people who like do-it-yourself crafts and creative pursuits, upcycling might be a more affordable option than purchasing new goods.

- **How to Initiate Upcycling**

- **Assess Your Materials:** Make a list of everything you own and think about how you might use it again. Seek out materials with unique qualities or that are still in good shape.

- **Organise Your Task:** Choose an inventive activity or concept for your repurposed resources. assemble any extra materials or equipment required for the makeover.

- **Try New Things and Be Creative:** Never be scared to try out various methods and designs. Upcycling provides a platform for individual expression and innovation.

5. Recycling and Upcycling Promotion

- **Involvement with the Community**

- **Education and Awareness:** Raise awareness of recycling and upcycling by holding workshops, events, and community activities. Inform people about the advantages these activities have for the economy and the environment.

- **Local Initiatives:** Encourage or take part in neighbourhood recycling initiatives, upcycling events, and creative reuse hubs that serve the community's needs and promote sustainable practices.

- **Teamwork and Creativity**

- **Partnerships:** Work with nearby companies, educational institutions, and groups to carry out upcycling and recycling projects. Exchange best practices, information, and resources to strengthen group initiatives.

- **Support Sustainable Brands:** Make purchases from businesses that place a high priority on upcycling and recycling. By giving these companies your support, you may encourage others to adopt sustainable business practices.

Reducing waste and advancing environmental sustainability are inextricably linked to recycling and upcycling. People may reduce waste, conserve resources, and contribute to a more sustainable future by being aware of and putting these habits into practice.

Whereas upcycling imaginatively repurposes objects to increase their life and worth, recycling uses industrial processing to turn wasted materials into new goods. Significant advantages of both strategies include social interaction, financial savings, and environmental preservation.

Adopting upcycling and recycling techniques calls for awareness, ingenuity, and community involvement. We can all contribute to a cleaner, greener, and more sustainable society by implementing these habits into our daily lives and inspiring others to do the same.

➤ Cutting Down on Single-Use Plastics: Towards a Sustainable Lifestyle

Single-use plastics, which are made to be used just once and then thrown away, are now commonplace in everyday life. Examples include straws, shopping bags, water bottles, and food containers. Even if they are practical, these products heavily pollute the environment, endangering ecosystems, wildlife, and public health. Reducing plastics that are used once is essential to the transition to a more sustainable future. This tutorial examines the problems with single-use plastics, the advantages of reduction, and workable methods for cutting back on plastic consumption in daily life.

1. Gaining Knowledge About Single-Use Plastics

- **Explanation and Illustrations**

Products constructed of plastic that are meant to be used just once before being thrown away are known as single-use plastics. Among them are:

- **Plastic Bags:** Frequently utilised for packing, retail purchases, and groceries.

- **Plastic Bottles:** These are used to hold liquids like juice, soda, and water.

- **Food Containers:** Contains disposable cutlery, plastic wrappers and takeaway containers.

- **Straws and Utensils:** Frequently utilised for convenience and in fast-food establishments.

- **Packaging Materials:** Packaging peanuts, plastic wrap, and bubble wrap are included.

- **Impact on the Environment**

- **Waste Accumulation:** Single-use plastics frequently wind up in landfills, where their decomposition might take centuries. They contribute to microplastic contamination as they decompose.

- **Ocean Pollution:** Plastics have a significant role in marine pollution, which negatively impacts ecosystems and marine life. Plastic garbage can harm or even kill animals if they swallow it or entangle themselves in it.

- **Resource Depletion:** Fossil fuels are needed in the production of single-use plastics, which adds to resource depletion and greenhouse gas emissions.

2. Advantages of Cutting Down on Single-Use Plastics

- **Preservation of the Environment**

- **Reduced Pollution:** We can conserve animals and preserve natural ecosystems by reducing the amount of plastic garbage we produce, which will also minimise the environmental impact on land and water.

- **Resource Conservation:** Cutting back on plastic consumption lowers the need for raw materials, protecting fossil fuels and lowering production-related energy costs.

- **Health Advantages**

- **Decreased Exposure to Toxins:** Plastics have the ability to contaminate food and drink with dangerous compounds, which may be hazardous to human health. Minimising the use of plastic reduces exposure to these poisons.

- **Cleaner Environments:** Streets, parks, and waterways are cleaner when there are fewer plastics around, improving general public health and quality of life.

- **Financial Reserves**

- **Cost-Effective Alternatives:** Stainless steel bottles and cloth bags are two reusable substitutes for single-use plastics that can save money over time.

- **Reduced Waste Management Costs:** Reducing plastic waste can help municipalities manage their waste more cheaply and ease the financial strain on their waste processing infrastructure.

3. Workable Plans for Cutting Down on Single-Use Plastics

- **Use Reusable Substitutes**

1. Sacks and Jars

- **Reusable Bags:** Instead of using plastic bags for your shopping, use cloth or mesh bags. Reusable bags come in a variety of sizes from many businesses, perfect for grocery and other purchases.

- **Reusable Containers:** For takeaway and food storage, use glass, metal or bamboo containers. These substitutes are reusable and long-lasting.

2. Glassware and Cutlery

- **Water Bottles:** Invest in a reusable bottle composed of glass, stainless steel, or plastic that doesn't contain BPA. As a result, fewer single-use plastic bottles are required.

- **silverware and Straws:** Use silicone, metal, or bamboo silverware and straws that can be reused. Keep them with you to cut down on throwaway choices.

- **Select Ecological Options**

1. Containerisation

- **Select Products with Minimal Packaging:** Make sure to choose products with eco-friendly or minimal packaging. Steer clear of anything packed in too much plastic or materials that cannot be recycled.

- **Buy in Bulk:** Buying goods in bulk lessens the demand for single-use plastic containers and cuts down on the quantity of packing.

2. Items for Personal Care

- **Select Plastic-Free Personal Care Products:** Reject plastic bottles and throwaway goods in favour of bar soap, shampoo bars and bamboo toothbrushes.

- **Refill Stations:** To cut down on plastic waste, use refill stations for cleaning supplies, shampoo, and conditioner.

- Encourage Plastic-Free Campaigns

1. Promote and Teach

- **Raise Awareness:** Inform friends, relatives, and neighbours about the dangers of single-use plastics and the advantages of reducing their use. Participate in neighbourhood cleanup initiatives and disseminate information on social media.

- **Legislation in Support:** Encourage the adoption of laws and rules aimed at reducing the use of plastic, such as those that prohibit the use of single-use plastic bags or provide incentives to companies who utilise sustainable practices.

2. Opt for Green Brands

- **Support Sustainable Businesses:** Make purchases from businesses that place a high value on sustainability and eco-friendly packaging. Seek out brands that make use of biodegradable, compostable, or recyclable materials.

- **Support Innovation:** Provide backing and capital to companies and startups who are coming up with creative ways to cut down on plastic waste and replace it with sustainable alternatives.

4. Surmounting Obstacles

- **Sustainability vs. Convenience**

- **Behavioural Change:** Making routine and habit changes may be necessary when switching from single-use plastics to reusable alternatives. To promote adoption, highlight the ease of usage and long-term advantages.

- **Accessibility:** Make sure that reasonably priced and easily accessible reusable alternatives are available. Speak up in favour of laws that encourage the production of sustainable goods.

- **Overall Modifications**

- **Corporate Responsibility:** Motivate companies to cut back on plastic packaging and implement sustainable practices. Encourage projects that advance environmental stewardship and business transparency.

- **Infrastructure Development:** Promote upgrades to waste management and recycling infrastructure to better manage plastic trash and aid in recycling initiatives.

A crucial first step towards a more sustainable future is reducing the usage of single-use plastics. People may greatly reduce their plastic footprint and aid in environmental conservation by using reusable alternatives, making thoughtful decisions, and endorsing eco-friendly projects.

Reducing single-use plastics improves health, saves money, and engages the community in addition to protecting the environment. Adopting these practices has significant benefits for both people and the environment, but it also demands dedication and teamwork.

Through proactive measures to reduce plastic consumption and motivating others to follow suit, we can jointly strive towards a world that is healthier, cleaner, and more sustainable.

Chapter 5

Green Cleaning: An Eco-Friendly Way to Make Your House Healthier

Using eco-friendly tools and methods, green cleaning places a high priority on human health, safety, and environmental sustainability. Conventional cleaning products frequently include dangerous chemicals that can have an adverse effect on the environment, human health, and indoor air quality. By choosing safer, more ecologically friendly options, green cleaning aims to address these problems. This article explores the fundamentals of green cleaning, its advantages, and doable actions to successfully apply green cleaning techniques.

1. Green cleaning principles

- **Non-Toxic Substances**

Ingredients used in the formulation of green cleaning solutions are less detrimental to the environment and human health. Harsh chemicals like ammonia, bleach, and phthalates are not used in these products, which can lead to breathing issues, skin irritation, and contamination of the environment.

- **Packaging that is Recyclable and Biodegradable**

Packaging for eco-friendly cleaning solutions is generally composed of recycled materials or biodegradable materials. This encourages the circular economy and lessens the negative effects of plastic waste on the environment.

- **Efficiency of Water and Energy**

Water and energy efficiency are also prioritised in green cleaning techniques. This involves choosing energy-efficient equipment that uses less electricity and cleaning techniques that utilise the least amount of water.

- **Diminished Ecological Damage**

By employing materials and techniques that are less detrimental to ecosystems and wildlife, green cleaning seeks to reduce the total environmental impact. This entails minimising the emission of volatile organic compounds (VOCs) and selecting goods that meet reliable environmental requirements for certification.

2. Green Cleaning's Advantages

- **Improved Indoor Air Quality**

Conventional cleaning supplies frequently emit volatile organic compounds (VOCs) and other airborne contaminants, exacerbating indoor air quality problems and respiratory disorders. Because they contain non-toxic components, green cleaning products contribute to better indoor air quality and a healthier living environment.

- **Decreased Contact with Dangerous Substances**

Using environmentally friendly cleaning supplies helps people limit their exposure to potentially dangerous chemicals. Pregnant women, families with small children, and anyone with allergies and respiratory disorders should pay special attention to this.

- **Preservation of the Environment**

Green cleaning techniques help protect the environment by cutting down on waste, pollution, and resource use. This promotes more general sustainability objectives and aids in the preservation of natural resources and ecosystems.

- **Economical Advantages**

Over time, green cleaning may also result in financial savings. Since many eco-friendly cleaning products are concentrated and need for fewer amounts, total costs may be lowered. Water and energy conservation measures can also reduce utility costs.

3. Eco-Friendly Cleaning Supplies

- **Do-it-yourself green cleaning solutions**

Making your own cleaning solutions is a great method to manage the components and implement green cleaning. Typical components of homemade cleansers are:

- **Vinegar:** Glass, counters, and bathrooms can all be cleaned with vinegar, a natural disinfectant and degreaser.

- **Baking Soda:** Baking soda is a mildly abrasive and odor-absorbing substance that can be used for deodorising and surface cleaning.

- **Lemon Juice:** Lemon juice can be used to clean and create a fresh aroma due to its inherent antibacterial qualities.

- **Sustainable Industrial Cleaners**

There are many commercial green cleaning products accessible for anyone who would rather use pre-made solutions. Seek for goods bearing certificates like these:

- **Green Seal:** An accreditation proving the product satisfies high performance and environmental requirements.

- **Environmental Choice:** An EcoLogo program accreditation attesting to the products' environmental responsibility.

- **EPA Safer Choice:** Goods bearing this mark have undergone evaluation by the Environmental Protection Agency of the United States and have been found to fulfil their standards for environmental and human health safety.

- **Eco-Friendly Cleaning Equipment**

Think about utilising eco-friendly cleaning instruments in addition to cleaning supplies, like:

- **Microfiber Cloths:** Paper towels and disposable wipes are less necessary when using reusable, very effective microfiber cloths to trap dust and debris.

- **Bamboo Brushes and Mops:** To help cut down on plastic waste, tools manufactured from sustainable materials like bamboo are available.

- **Recycled or Biodegradable Sponges:** You can compost or recycle sponges made of natural fibres or recycled materials.

4. Eco-Friendly Cleaning Methods

- **Methods of Cleaning**

- **Dry Dusting:** To collect dust without using chemical sprays, use a microfiber cloth. As a result, less dust and allergens are released into the atmosphere.

- **Spot Cleaning:** Take care of spills and stains right away to avoid requiring further cleaning. This may lessen the need for harsh cleaning agents.

- **Appropriate Ventilation:** To minimise the concentration of any airborne contaminants and to facilitate the drying process, make sure adequate ventilation is in place during cleaning.

- **Efficiency of Water and Energy**

- **Use Energy-Efficient Equipment:** To save energy, select cleaning supplies and apparatus that have earned an ENERGY STAR® rating.

- **Reduce Water Use:** Avoid running the taps while cleaning, and use water-saving mops and cleaning equipment.

- **Minimising Waste**

Reuse cleaning cloths and utensils and recycle packaging wherever you can to adhere to the Reduce, Reuse, Recycle philosophy.

- **Bulk Purchasing:** buy cleaning supplies in large quantities to cut down on packaging waste and buy frequency.

5. Putting Green Cleaning Into Practice at Home

- **Examine Your Cleaning Supplies**

Assess the cleaning supplies you currently own first. Look for any that come in non-recyclable packaging or contain dangerous substances. Swap these out for more environmentally friendly options.

- **Inform Members of the Household**

Teach every family member the advantages of utilising eco-friendly products and green cleaning techniques.

Urge everyone to embrace the shift to greener techniques and develop sustainable cleaning habits.

- **Establish a Green Cleaning Schedule**

Create a cleaning schedule that uses green cleaning supplies and methods. Establish precise cleaning activities and timetables to guarantee efficiency and consistency.

- **Observe and Modify**

To increase efficacy and efficiency, assess and modify your green cleaning procedures on a regular basis. Keep up with new developments in eco-friendly cleaning supplies and methods, and adjust as necessary.

6. Overcoming Typical Obstacles

- **Issues with Effectiveness**

It's possible that some individuals believe conventional cleaning products are more effective than green ones. Nonetheless, a lot of environmentally friendly products are made to function on par with or better than traditional cleansers. Try out several items and techniques to see which suits your needs the best.

- **Expense Points to Take into Account**

Despite the fact that some green cleaning products may cost more up front, their concentrated formulations and extended shelf lives sometimes make them more affordable over time. An affordable option can also be to do things yourself.

- **Accessibility**

It could be hard to get environmentally friendly products in some places. Seek out local health food stores and internet merchants who provide eco-friendly cleaning solutions. As a convenient and affordable substitute, think about creating your own cleaning solutions.

Green cleaning is an environmentally friendly, sustainable way to keep your house clean and healthy. People can select for eco-friendly products, biodegradable packaging, and energy-saving techniques to support environmental aims and create a better living environment.

Choosing environmentally friendly products, utilising sustainable cleaning supplies, and implementing effective cleaning methods are all part of putting green cleaning practices into practice. People may contribute to a cleaner, greener future by reducing their ecological footprint and raising awareness through educated decision-making.

Making the switch to green cleaning has major advantages for the environment, human health, and long-term financial savings, but it also demands dedication and education. A vital first step in making your home healthier and more sustainable is adopting green cleaning techniques.

➢ DIY Natural Cleaning Solutions

A clean and healthy house can be maintained with natural cleaning solutions instead of the harsh chemicals present in many commercial cleaning products. You may make inexpensive, safe, and environmentally friendly cleaning solutions for your family and the environment by combining ordinary household materials with them. This article covers many natural cleaning solutions that may be made at home, their advantages, and useful advice on how to make and use them.

1. Advantages of Doing Your Own Natural Cleaning

- **Improved Indoor Air Quality**

The volatile organic compounds (VOCs) and other dangerous chemicals present in traditional cleaning products are typically avoided by using natural cleaning solutions. By enhancing indoor air quality, allergies and respiratory problems are less likely to occur.

- **Environmentally Sustainable**

In comparison to synthetic chemicals, materials used in do-it-yourself cleaning solutions are frequently biodegradable and have a smaller environmental impact. This lessens waste production and pollution.

- **Economical**

Generally speaking, homemade cleaning solutions are less expensive than items from the market. Baking soda, vinegar, and lemon juice are inexpensive and widely accessible ingredients.

- **Adaptable**

You can customise homemade cleaning solutions by adding smells or changing the solution's strength to fit your unique requirements and tastes.

2. Vital Components for Do-It-Yourself Cleaning Solutions

- **Vinegar**

- **Properties:** Vinegar has natural deodorising and disinfecting properties. Its acidic qualities aid in the dissolution of dirt, grease, and mineral deposits.

- **Uses:** May be applied to floors, counters, and glass.

- **Soda Baking**

- **Properties:** Baking soda has deodorising and mild abrasive properties. It aids in cleaning surfaces and removing smells.

- **Uses:** Works well on stovetops, bathtubs, and sinks.

- **Juice from Lemons**

- **Properties:** Lemon juice naturally possesses antiviral and antibacterial qualities. It also functions as a natural deodoriser and bleach.

- **Uses:** Effective at getting rid of stains, cleaning, and introducing a new aroma.

- **Castille Soap**

- **Features:** Castile soap is a vegetable-based soap that is mild on surfaces and biodegradable. It works well for cleaning and chopping oil.

- **Uses:** Excellent as a basis for different cleaning solutions and for all-purpose cleaning.

- **Vital Oils**

- **Properties:** Essential oils with antibacterial qualities, such as tea tree, lavender, and peppermint, can infuse cleaning solutions with pleasant aromas.

- **Uses:** Added to cleaning solutions for aroma and therapeutic properties.

3. Do-it-yourself Organic Cleaning Products

- **All-Utility Cleaner**

Components:
One cup of distilled white vinegar, one cup of water, and ten drops of essential oil (such as tea tree, lemon, or lavender)

Guidelines
1. Fill a spray bottle with equal parts vinegar and water.
2. Include the essential oil and thoroughly mix.
3. Apply a mist and use a cloth to clean the surfaces.

Uses: Countertops, tiles, and other hard surfaces can all be cleaned with this multipurpose cleaner.

- **Glass Cleaner**

Components:

One cup of distilled white vinegar, one cup of water, and one tablespoon of cornflour

Guidelines:

1. In a spray bottle, combine all ingredients.
Shake thoroughly before using.
3. For a streak-free shine, spray on glass surfaces and wipe with a microfiber cloth.

Uses: Ideal for wiping off glass surfaces, mirrors, and windows.

- **Soda Scrub Baking**

Components:
- One-half cup baking soda
- One tablespoon of liquid Castile soap - 1/4 cup of water

Guidelines:

1. Make a paste by combining the baking soda and water.

2. Include the Castile soap and blend thoroughly.

3. Use a sponge or towel to scrub the surface after applying the paste.

4. Give it a good rinse.

Uses: Works well for cleaning stovetops, bathtubs, and sinks.

- **Mop the Floor**

Components:

- 1/4 cup baking soda - 1/4 cup distilled white vinegar
- One gallon of hot water

Guidelines:

1. Stir the baking soda and vinegar into the heated water.

2. Use the solution to mop the floors, making sure to squeeze out any extra liquid from the mop.

Uses: Effective on vinyl, tile, and linoleum floors. On hardwood floors, stay away from utilising as too much moisture might harm the wood.

- **Cleaning Supplies for Bathrooms**

Components:

- One-half cup baking soda
- Ten drops of essential oil (optional) - 1/4 cup distilled white vinegar - 1/4 cup water

Guidelines:

1. In a bowl, mix the vinegar and baking soda.
2. To make a paste, add water.
3. Use on tile, tub and sink surfaces in bathrooms.
4. Use a sponge to scrub, then give it a good rinse.

Uses: Assists in thoroughly cleaning and deodorising washroom surfaces.

- **Refresher for Fabric**

Components:

- 1/4 cup vodka or rubbing alcohol - 1 cup water
- Ten drops of essential oil (peppermint or lavender, for example)

Guidelines:

Mix all the ingredients together in a spray bottle.

Shake thoroughly before using.

3. To revive and deodorise materials, such as drapes and upholstery, lightly mist.

Uses: Great for reviving clothes and getting rid of smells.

4. Advice on Using Homemade Natural Cleaning Products

- **Conduct a Test First**

Any new cleaning solution should always be tested on a small, discrete area before being used on a larger surface. This makes it more likely that the solution won't damage or discolour anything.

- **Adequate Storage**

Homemade cleaning supplies should be kept out of direct sunlight and heat sources in labelled containers. To keep the solutions' efficacy, make sure the containers are firmly sealed.

- **Appropriate Use**

To get the best results, use the recommended cleaning products, including non-abrasive sponges or microfiber towels, and follow the directions provided with each cleaning solution.

- **Try New Things and Modify**

To make your cleaning solutions unique to your requirements and tastes, feel free to experiment with different component combinations and essential oils.

An economical and environmentally responsible substitute for traditional cleaning chemicals are homemade natural cleaning solutions. You can make inexpensive, safe, and environmentally friendly cleaning solutions for your home that work wonders for the environment by using common household components. Adopting these natural cleaning techniques encourages sustainable living while improving indoor air quality and lowering chemical exposure.

Using homemade natural cleaning products requires a dedication to making better decisions and being environmentally conscious. You can keep your house fresh and clean while leaving as little of an environmental impact as possible with a little imagination and trial and error.

➢ Reusable Cleaning Supplies: Sustainable Home Options with Eco-Friendly Substitutes

Using reusable cleaning products is a practical method to cut waste and environmental impact when living a greener lifestyle. Reusable tools, as opposed to single-use or throwaway ones, are made to be used repeatedly and have advantages for the environment and the economy. This article looks at different reusable cleaning products, their benefits, and how to use them for a more environmentally friendly home.

1. Benefits of Cleaning Tools That Can Be Reused

- **Reducing Waste**

Reusable cleaning supplies reduce the quantity of garbage dumped in landfills. Selecting reusable products lessens the need for throwaway goods like paper towels, which add to pollution in the environment.

- **Economical Advantages**

Reusable instruments may require a larger initial investment, but over time, their cost-effectiveness usually increases. The necessity for frequent repurchasing is lessened by the extended lifespan and ease of cleaning and maintenance of reusable objects.

- **The Effect on the Environment**

Compared to single-use items, reusable cleaning equipment has a smaller environmental impact because they are often constructed from recycled or sustainable materials. You may lessen the need for new resources and promote sustainable practices by selecting eco-friendly materials.

- **Sturdiness and Effectiveness**

Reusable cleaning equipment of the highest calibre are made to last. They have more cleaning power and lifespan than some disposable options and are frequently made to tolerate repeated usage.

2. Sorts of Cleaning Tools That Can Be Reused

- **Microfiber Towels**

Features:

- **Material:** Polyester and polyamide are examples of synthetic fibres.
- **Features:** Absorbent to the max, efficient at collecting dust and debris, and kind to surfaces.
- **Uses:** Excellent alternative to chemical cleaners for cleaning windows, counters, and electronics.

Features:
- **Reusable:** May be cleaned and used again.
- **Effective:** Requires less cleaning solution and water than conventional clothes.

Care Advice:
- **Washing:** To prevent lint accumulation, wash microfiber cloths apart from regular laundry. Avoid fabric softeners and use a mild detergent instead.
- **Drying:** To protect the fibres, air dry or tumble dry on low heat.

- **Easily Reusable Mop**

Features:

- **Material:** Washable cotton or microfiber are commonly used to make mop heads.
- **Design:** A lot of models have machine-washable and detachable mop heads.

Advantages:
- **Effective Cleaning:** Offers comprehensive cleaning and works with a variety of cleaning agents.
- **Resilient:** minimises the need for replacements and throwaway mop pads.

Maintenance Advice:
- **Rinsing:** After using the mop, rinse and wring out the head. As directed by the manufacturer, give it a regular wash.
- **Storage:** To stop mildew from growing, let the mop head air dry fully before storing.

- Sponge Reusables

Features:

- **Material:** Reusable, washable fibres, either natural or synthetic.
- **Design:** While some sponges are constructed of materials that can be composted, such cellulose, others are built to last.

Advantages:
- **Economical:** reusable for several uses before needing replacement.
- **Eco-Friendly:** Minimises the requirement for single-use sponges.

Care Instructions:
- **Cleaning:** Boil, microwave, or run your sponges through the dishwasher to completely rinse them after each use.
- **Replacement:** When sponges begin to show wear or deterioration, replace them.

- **Cleaners with refillable bottles**

Features:

- **Material:** Glass or sturdy polymers that may be filled with cleaning agents are used to make this product.
- **Design:** Frequently featuring pump motors or spray nozzles.

Features:
- **Decreased Waste:** Gets rid of the requirement for containers for cleaning products that are only used once.
- **Available:** enables the use of DIY or large-scale cleaning products.

Taking Care of It
- **Cleaning:** To avoid contamination, give bottles a thorough wash before refilling.
- **Labelling:** To prevent confusion, clearly mark bottles with their contents.

- **Wooden or bamboo scrub brushes**

Features:
- **Material:** Bristles made of recycled or natural fibres, handles made of bamboo or other sustainable woods.

- **Design:** available in a variety of forms, including as toilet, scrub, and dish brushes.

Advantages:
- **Environmentally friendly:** Wood and bamboo are renewable materials with minimal effect on the environment.
- **Sturdy:** Designed to endure and tolerate frequent use.

Care Instructions:
- **Cleaning:** After using a brush, properly rinse it and let it air dry.
- **Upkeep:** If any parts or brushes become worn down or broken, replace them.

3. Making Use of Reusable Cleaning Equipment

- **Proceed Gradually**

Start by switching out one or two disposable cleaning tools for ones that may be reused. Replace paper towels with microfiber cloths, for instance, and add more reusable things gradually as needed.

- **Inform Members of the Household**

Teach everyone in the house the advantages of using reusable cleaning supplies and how to use them properly. Urge them to adhere to maintenance rules and take part in the transfer.

- **Establish a Cleaning Schedule**

Include reusable cleaning supplies in your regimen. Make sure every tool is conveniently accessible for frequent usage and has a designated storage area.

- **Continual Upkeep**

Follow the manufacturer's instructions for cleaning and maintaining your reusable tools. The tools' lifespan can be increased and their functionality can be guaranteed with proper maintenance.

- **Observe and Modify**

Your reusable tools should be evaluated for effectiveness and adjusted as necessary. If some tools are not working as you would want, you might want to test other brands or options.

4. Dealing with Typical Issues

- **Original Expense**

Reusable cleaning supplies may initially cost more than their disposable counterparts. But when assessing the investment, take into account the long-term savings and environmental advantages.

- **Upkeep and Sanitisation**

Reusable tool lifetime and performance depend on regular cleaning and maintenance. To preserve performance, strictly follow the care recommendations and take quick action as necessary.

- **Accessibility**

It could be difficult to get high-quality reusable cleaning tools in some places. Seek out internet merchants and niche shops that carry a variety of environmentally friendly cleaning supplies.

An eco-friendly and sustainable home must have reusable cleaning supplies. You can keep a tidy and useful living area and help the environment at the same time by choosing goods that minimise waste and encourage ecologically friendly habits.

Adopting eco-friendly habits and cutting back on single-use items are prerequisites for using reusable cleaning tools in your house. Reusable cleaning products can improve your routine and encourage a more sustainable lifestyle with careful selection, upkeep, and intelligent application.

➢ Eco-Friendly Brands: Leading the Way for a Sustainable Future

Growing consumer knowledge of environmental issues has led to a demand for brands that emphasise eco-friendliness and sustainability. Brands that are environmentally conscious are dedicated to minimising their influence on the environment, use sustainable products, and encouraging moral behaviour. This guide showcases several well-known environmentally conscious companies from a range of sectors, highlighting their dedication to sustainability and offering ideas for choosing more environmentally friendly products.

1. Green Cleaning Product Brands

- **Technique**

Overview: Method is renowned for its dedication to creating cleaning solutions that are safe for the environment by using recycled packaging and biodegradable components.

- **Sustainability Focus:** Offers a variety of products, ranging from hand soaps to all-purpose cleansers, using non-toxic, plant-based components.

- **Notable Products:** Method Antibacterial Bathroom Cleaner, Method All-Purpose Cleaner.

- **Generation Seven**

Overview: Seventh Generation provides a broad range of environmentally friendly personal care and household cleaning products.

- **Sustainability Focus:** Places a strong emphasis on using recyclable packaging, carbon-neutral shipping, and plant-based products.

- **Prominent Items:** Seventh Generation Laundry Detergent, Seventh Generation Disinfecting Wipes.

- **Recover**

Overview: Ecover is committed to making environmentally friendly cleaning products that work well.

- **Sustainability Focus:** Makes use of mineral and plant-based ingredients, biodegradable recipes, and recyclable packaging.

- **Notable Products:** Ecover Bathroom Cleaner, Ecover Zero Laundry Detergent.

2. Brands of Eco-Friendly Personal Care Products

- **Dr. Bronner's**

Overview: Dr. Bronner's is well-known for its organic Castile soap, which is used for a variety of purposes, as well as its dedication to fair trade and ecological sustainability.

- **Sustainability Focus:** All ingredients are fair trade and certified organic; 100% post-consumer recycled plastic is used for packaging.

- **Notable Products:** Dr. Bronner's Organic Lip Balm and Pure-Castile Liquid Soap.

- **2. Intense**

Overview: Lush is renowned for its high ethical standards and freshly created personal care products.

- **Emphasis on Sustainability:** emphasises the use of natural and ethically sourced materials, minimal packaging, and cruelty-free procedures.

- **Notable Items:** Lush Fresh Face Masks, Lush Shampoo Bars.

- **The Burt's Bees Company**

Overview: With an emphasis on sustainability and environmental stewardship, Burt's Bees provides a selection of natural personal care products.

- **Sustainability Focus:** Makes use of natural materials, environmentally friendly packaging, and takes steps to lessen its carbon footprint.

- **Notable Products:** Burt's Bees Facial Cleansing Towelettes and Beeswax Lip Balm.

3. Brands of Eco-Friendly Clothing and Accessories

- Patagonia

Overview: Renowned for its inventive methods and environmental activism, Patagonia is a pioneer in environmentally conscious outdoor clothing and equipment.

- **Emphasis on Sustainability:** utilises organic cotton, recyclable materials, and ethical labour standards.

provides a repair program to increase the longevity of its products.

- **Prominent Items:** Patagonia Nano Puff Jacket, Patagonia Better Sweater.

- **TOMS**

Overview: TOMS is renowned for their environmentally friendly footwear and socially conscious company practices.

- **Emphasis on Sustainability:** uses eco-friendly materials—like recycled plastic and organic cotton—and contributes to a number of charity causes.

- **Notable Products:** Earthwise Collection and TOMS Classics.

- **Reorganisation**

Overview: Reformation specialises in lessening the environmental impact of its fashionable, eco-friendly clothing.

- **Sustainability Focus:** Makes use of environmentally friendly materials, conserves water and energy, and provides a garment take-back program.

- Notable Items: Reformation Denim and Dresses.

4. Brands of Green Kitchen and Home Products

- **Grove Collaborative, Inc.**

Overview: Grove Collaborative is dedicated to sustainability and offers a large selection of environmentally friendly personal care and household items.

- **Sustainability Focus:** Offers natural ingredient items, recyclable packaging, and a range of environmentally friendly brands.

- **Notable Products:** Paper products and cleaning supplies made by Grove Collaborative.

- **The Bee's Wrap**

Overview: Bee's Wrap uses organic cotton and beeswax to provide a sustainable substitute for plastic wrap.

- **Sustainability Focus:** Encourages compostable and reusable food storage options to cut down on waste from single-use plastics.

- **Notable Products:** Sandwich wraps and reusable food wraps made by Bee's Wrap.

- **Organiser**

Overview: As an eco-friendly and reusable substitute for plastic bags, Stasher manufactures silicone storage bags.

- **Sustainability Focus:** Encourages the reduction of single-use plastics and uses food-grade, non-toxic silicone.

- **Notable Products:** Stasher Stand-Up Bags, Silicone Storage Bags.

5. Brands of Green Technology

- **Fairphone**

Overview: Fairphone is dedicated to making sustainable and moral cellphones, emphasising fair labour standards and recyclable components.

- **Sustainability Focus:** Gives top priority to materials free from conflicts, modular designs for simple maintenance, and open supply chains.

- **Notable Products:** Fairphone Accessories, Fairphone 4.

- **Electric vehicle**

Overview: With a focus on lowering dependency on fossil fuels, Tesla is at the forefront of sustainable energy and electric car technology.

- **Sustainability Focus:** Works to accelerate the shift to sustainable energy by developing solar energy products, energy storage systems, and electric vehicles.

- **Significant Items:** Powerwall, Model 3 Tesla.

- **Generation Seven**

Overview: Seventh Generation is well-known for its assortment of environmentally friendly products, but it also offers tech items that prioritise sustainability.

- **Sustainability Focus:** Encourages environmental advocacy, supports carbon offsetting, and makes use of eco-friendly materials.

- **Notable Products:** Cleaning products and seventh-generation recycled paper products.

6. Endorsing Green Brands

- **Investigation and Confirmation**

Examine a company's certifications, sustainability policies, and product ingredients before selecting an eco-friendly brand. To verify authenticity, look for third-party certifications such as Fair Trade, Organic, or Cradle to Cradle.

- **Awareness and Advocacy**

Give your support to companies who actively raise awareness of environmental issues and take part in community projects. This boosts their efforts and motivates more businesses to implement sustainable practices.

- **Conscientious Buying**

Think about how your purchases will affect you overall, taking into account packing and shipping methods. Select brands that use environmentally friendly packaging materials and reduce waste.

By providing items that lessen their impact on the environment and encourage ethical behaviour, eco-friendly firms are setting the standard for a more sustainable future. By endorsing these goods, you not only help the environment but also inspire other businesses to do the same.

Adopting environmentally friendly companies in a variety of sectors, such as personal care and cleaning supplies, clothing, and technology, enables you to make thoughtful decisions that improve your house and the environment. These companies are leading the way towards a future that is healthier and more sustainable through their unwavering innovation and dedication to sustainability.

Chapter 6

Eco-Friendly Gardening: Fostering a Greener Tomorrow

Sustainable gardening is a practice based on resource conservation, environmental responsibility, and comprehensive land management, not just a fad. You can design a garden that encourages biodiversity, lessens waste, and supports regional ecosystems by using sustainable gardening practices. This article provides helpful guidance for growing a greener, more resilient garden by examining the fundamental ideas and techniques of sustainable gardening.

1. Gaining Knowledge About Sustainable Gardening

1.1. Purpose and Objectives

The goal of sustainable gardening is to design a green space that strikes a balance between ecological health and productivity. The main objectives are to:

- **Minimise Environmental Impact:** Cut back on waste, synthetic chemicals, and non-renewable resource usage.

- **Improve Biodiversity:** Promote a wide variety of flora and fauna to maintain the stability of ecosystems.

- **Conserve Resources:** To maintain the health of your garden over time, adopt techniques for conserving water and soil.

- **Support Local Food Systems:** Grow food locally to cut down on transportation-related carbon footprints.

1.2. Crucial Ideas

- **Soil Health:** Make natural practices and additions a priority to improve soil fertility.

- **Water Management:** Reduce runoff and conserve water by using effective watering methods.

- **Plant Selection:** Select native plants that can withstand dryness and grow well in your area.

- **Waste Reduction:** Reduce waste by using recycling and composting techniques.

2. Management and Health of the Soil

2.1. Composting and Organic Matter

- **Organic Matter:** To enhance soil structure, water retention, and fertility, add organic matter such as compost, aged manure, or leaf mulch.

- **Composting:** To recycle yard trash, food scraps and other organic wastes, set up a compost bin or pile. Composting adds vital nutrients to the soil while decreasing waste.

2.2. Amendments and Soil Testing

- **Soil Testing:** Test the soil to determine its pH, nitrogen levels, and other characteristics. Knowing the makeup of your soil will help you choose the right amendments.

- **Natural Amendments:** To improve soil fertility without using artificial chemicals, apply natural fertilisers like bone meal, blood meal, or green manure.

2.3. Control of Erosion

- **Cover Crops:** To prevent soil erosion, enhance soil structure, and replenish organic matter, plant cover crops like rye or clover.

- **Terracing and Mulching:** To prevent soil erosion and preserve moisture, use terracing on slopes and apply mulch.

3. Water Management and Conservation

3.1. Watering Methods That Work

- **Drip Irrigation:** To reduce evaporation and runoff, use a drip irrigation system to supply water straight to plant roots.

- **Rainwater Harvesting:** Use barrels or cisterns to gather rainwater for watering gardens. This procedure lowers water expenses while conserving tap water.

3.2. Plants Resistant to Drought

- **Native Plants:** Select native plants that need less water and upkeep and are acclimated to the local climate.

- **Drought-Tolerant Varieties:** Choose plant cultivars that can tolerate dry spells and periods of low precipitation.

3.3. Methods for Conserving Water

- **Mulching:** Use mulch around plants to control temperature, keep soil moist, and keep weeds at bay.

- **Timetable for Watering:** In order to reduce evaporation and guarantee efficient water usage, water plants in the early morning or late at night.

4. Biodiversity and Plant Selection

4.1. Plants That Are Native and Adaptive

- **Native Plants:** Choose native plants that are appropriate for your garden's environment and that benefit the local fauna. Generally speaking, they require less pesticides, fertilisers, and water.

- **Adaptive Plants:** Select plants that are suitable for the particular microclimate, kind of soil, and exposure levels in your garden.

4.2. Plants That Are Good Pollinators

- **Flowering Plants:** To draw pollinators such as bees and butterflies, cultivate a range of flowering plants. Coneflowers, sunflowers, and lavender are great options for plants.

- **Habitat Creation:** To maintain pollinator populations, create habitats like butterfly roosts, bee hotels, and native plants.

4.3. Planting with a Friend

- **Beneficial Pairings:** To improve plant productivity and health, use companion planting. For instance, planting marigolds alongside tomatoes can aid in insect deterrence.

- **Crop Rotation:** Turn your crops once a year to keep the soil from getting too thin and to lower your risk of pests and illnesses.

5. Recycling and Waste Reduction

5.1. The process of composting

- **Kitchen Scraps:** To cut down on kitchen waste and make nutrient-rich compost for your garden, compost eggshells, vegetable peels, and fruit scraps.

- **Yard Waste:** To recycle yard waste and enhance soil health, add grass clippings, leaves and prunings to your compost pile or bin.

5.2. Materials Recycled

- **Garden Containers:** For planters and garden beds, use repurposed wood, pallets, or old containers.

- **Garden Tools:** To increase the life of your garden tools, choose those composed of sustainable or recycled materials and give them regular upkeep.

5.3. Cutting Down on Plastic Use

- **Avoid Single-Use Plastics:** Use less plastic gardening tools and choose compostable or biodegradable containers instead.

- **Reusables:** To cut down on plastic waste, use reusable irrigation systems, plant ties, and garden coverings.

6. Techniques and Practices for Sustainability

6.1. IPM, or Integrated Pest Management

- **Biological Controls:** Employ nematodes or ladybirds, two naturally occurring predators, to manage pests. Refrain from using broad-spectrum pesticides as they may damage helpful insects.

- **Cultural Practices:** To lessen insect issues, use techniques like crop rotation, appropriate spacing, and cleanliness.

6.2. Management of Organic Pests

- **Natural Remedies:** To handle garden pests without using hazardous chemicals, use organic pest management techniques like neem oil, insecticidal soap, or garlic sprays.

- **Physical Barriers:** To shield plants from insects and wildlife, erect barriers like netting or row covers.

6.3. Energy-Saving Techniques

- **Solar Power:** To save energy and promote sustainable energy sources, use solar-powered tools, irrigation systems, and garden lights.

- **Greenhouse Management:** Reduce energy consumption in greenhouses by implementing energy-saving techniques like passive solar heating and ventilation systems.

A complete approach to creating a garden that balances with the environment and saves resources is known as sustainable gardening. Gardeners may create dynamic, environmentally friendly landscapes that are advantageous to the community and the environment by concentrating on soil health, water conservation, plant selection, and waste reduction.

Using sustainable gardening techniques improves your garden's resilience and productivity while also lessening its ecological impact. Whether you're creating a new garden or making changes to an old one, following these guidelines will make gardening more pleasurable, sustainable, and ecologically conscious.

Sustainable gardening provides a route to a greener future where gardens flourish in balance with the environment and improve the health of our world with careful design and dedication.

➢ Organic Gardening: Using Natural Techniques to Nurture Nature

Using natural methods and resources to cultivate plants instead of artificial chemicals or genetically modified organisms is the focus of organic gardening, which is a sustainable gardening strategy. Organic gardening cultivates better, more nutrient-dense food while promoting environmental stewardship through an emphasis on soil health, biodiversity, and ecological balance. This guide offers helpful advice for creating a flourishing, environmentally friendly garden while summarising the main ideas, techniques, and advantages of organic gardening.

1. Organic Gardening Principles

1.1. Health of Soil

- **Creating Fertile Soil:** The foundation of organic farming is healthy soil. Rich in organic content, healthy soil improves in structure, fertility, and water-holding ability. To improve and preserve soil health, use cover crops, aged manure, and compost.

- **Eschewing Synthetic Chemicals:** With organic gardening, synthetic pesticides and fertilisers are avoided. Rather, it depends on biological pest management and natural amendments to keep the soil healthy and the plants vigorous.

1.2. Biodiversity

- **Diverse Planting:** Plant a range of plants to establish an ecosystem that is balanced and home to birds, insects, and other wildlife. Diversity strengthens the resilience of gardens and lowers the chance of pest and disease outbreaks.

- **Companion Planting:** To increase plant productivity and health, use companion planting strategies. For instance, putting marigolds close to tomatoes can help keep pests away, while planting beans nearby can support nearby plants by fixing nitrogen in the soil.

1.3. Care of the Environment

- **Resource Conservation:** Water and energy conservation are key components of organic growing. To save water and cut down on waste, use techniques like mulching and drip watering.

- **Minimising Waste:** Reuse, recycle, and reduce materials as much as you can. Compost garden and kitchen leftovers to improve soil quality and reduce waste going to landfills.

2. Organic Gardening Soil Management

2.1. The Process of Composting

- **Making Compost:** An essential step in organic farming is composting. Gather yard debris, cooking leftovers, and other organic materials to make compost that is high in nutrients. Composting enhances the fertility, structure, and moisture-holding capacity of soil.

- **Composting Techniques:** Select from a variety of composting techniques, including pile composting, bin composting, and vermicomposting (which uses worms). Every technique has advantages and may be customised to the size and requirements of your garden.

2.2. Amendments to Soil

- **Organic Fertilisers:** To provide plants the vital nutrients they need, apply organic fertilisers like kelp meal, fish emulsion, or bone meal. Slow nitrogen release from organic fertilisers lowers runoff danger and improves soil health over the long term.

- **Green Manure:** To enrich the soil with organic matter and nutrients, use cover crops or green manure crops like rye or clover. Green manure crops also aid in weed suppression and erosion prevention.

2.3. Preservation of Soil

- **Mulching:** Cover the soil's surface with organic mulch, such as wood chips, straw, or leaves. Mulching aids in controlling soil temperature, weed suppression, and moisture retention.

- **Erosion Control:** To stop soil erosion and safeguard the health of the soil, use erosion control techniques like terracing or growing ground coverings.

3. Management of Pests and Diseases

3.1. IPM, or Integrated Pest Management

- **Biological Controls:** To manage garden pests, make use of beneficial insects and natural predators. Aphids are the prey of ladybirds and lacewings, whereas caterpillars are the focus of parasitic wasps.

- **Physical Barriers:** To shield plants from pests and diseases, use physical barriers like nets or row covers. Barriers are very useful against birds and insects.

3.2. Management of Organic Pests

- **Natural Remedies:** Manage pests with organic pest management techniques like garlic sprays, neem oil, or insecticidal soap. When compared to synthetic pesticides, these remedies cause less damage to the environment and beneficial organisms.

- **Cultural Customs:** Adopt cultural techniques, such as crop rotation, appropriate spacing, and routine monitoring for early indications of infestations, that lessen insect problems.

3.3. Preventing Illnesses

- **Disease-Resistant kinds:** To lower the danger of plant illnesses, select disease-resistant plant kinds and maintain appropriate garden cleanliness. Take out and discard any contaminated plant debris right away.

- **Soil Management:** To increase air circulation and lower the risk of bacterial and fungal illnesses, keep your soil healthy and refrain from overloading your plants.

4. The Management of Water

4.1. Watering Methods That Work

- **Drip Irrigation:** To reduce evaporation and runoff, use a drip irrigation system to supply water straight to plant roots. Drip irrigation is very effective and adaptable to each plant's requirements.

- **Collecting Rainwater:** Gather and hold rainwater to irrigate gardens. Cisterns and rain barrels are two ways to lower water bills and conserve tap water.

4.2. Techniques to Conserve Water

- **Mulching:** To keep soil moisture in plants and lessen the need for regular watering, apply mulch around them. Mulch also aids in controlling soil temperature and weed suppression.

- **Watering Schedule:** To reduce evaporation and guarantee efficient water use, water plants in the early morning or late evening.

4.3. Controlling Soil Moisture

- **Soil Testing:** To prevent over- or under-watering, test the moisture content of the soil on a regular basis. Adapt your watering techniques to the soil's moisture content and the local climate.

- **Watering Methodologies:** Employ water-saving strategies when watering, such as sparingly and deeply watering to promote deep root development.

5. Ecological Methods

5.1. Gardening with Minimal Energy Use

- **Solar Power:** To save energy and promote sustainable energy sources, use solar power for equipment, irrigation systems, and lights in gardens.

- **Greenhouse Management:** Reduce energy consumption in greenhouses by implementing energy-saving techniques like passive solar heating and ventilation systems.

5.2. Preservation of Resources

- **Recycling:** To cut waste and promote sustainability, recycle garden items like plant pots and gardening tools.

- **Reusable Supplies:** To reduce plastic waste, choose reusable gardening tools like compostable garden bags and cloth plant ties.

5.3. Involvement with the Community

- **Educational Outreach:** Use social media, community gardens, and workshops to educate others about organic gardening. Educating people makes a network of environmentally conscious gardeners and helps to encourage sustainable practices.

- **Local Support:** To improve the regional food system and lessen its negative environmental effects, support nearby and organic farms, garden centres, and suppliers.

6. Advantages of Gardening in Organic Soil

6.1. Advantages for the Environment

- **Reduced Chemical Use:** By doing away with the need for artificial fertilisers and pesticides, organic farming lowers pollution and safeguards water supplies.

- **Soil Health:** By enhancing the fertility, biodiversity, and soil structure through organic activities, ecosystems and plant development are enhanced.

6.2. Advantages to Health

- **Nutrient-Rich Food:** Food grown organically is free of artificial additives and genetically modified organisms, which may result in food with a higher nutritious content.

- **Reduced Exposure:** By lowering exposure to dangerous chemicals, organic gardening methods improve customers' and gardeners' general health and wellbeing.

6.3. Financial Gains

- **Cost Savings:** By lowering the need for synthetic inputs and fostering self-sufficiency through homegrown produce, organic gardening can be financially advantageous over time.

- **Market Opportunities:** Gardeners who sell their food may gain financially because organic produce frequently fetches higher prices in the market.

Growing food and developing plants can be done in an environmentally responsible and satisfying way with organic gardening. Gardeners may build vibrant, environmentally friendly gardens that benefit people and the environment by emphasising soil health, biodiversity, and sustainable methods.

Using organic gardening practices improves your garden's sustainability and quality while also promoting environmental conservation. Adopting organic gardening methods can lead to a more robust, healthy, and environmentally friendly gardening experience, regardless of your level of skill.

You may reap the numerous advantages of a thriving, environmentally friendly garden while also making a positive contribution to a more sustainable future with careful design and a dedication to organic practices.

➢ Native and Vertical Plants: Eco-Friendly and Space-Saving Ways to Improve Your Garden

The sustainability, aesthetic appeal, and usability of your garden can all be greatly improved by adding native and vertical plants. While vertical gardening maximises space and provides visual interest, native plants are more beneficial to the environment and require less care. This tutorial examines the benefits of vertical gardening and native plants, offering helpful advice on how to incorporate both into your landscape design.

1. Native Plants: Benefits to the Environment and Beauty

1.1. Comprehending Indigenous Plants

- **Definition****: Native plants are species that are found naturally in a particular area or habitat and have evolved throughout time to adapt to the particular environmental conditions there. They consist of locally native floral plants, grasses, shrubs, and trees.

- **Advantages:** Native plants are hardy and low-maintenance since they are adapted to the soil, climate, and water conditions of the area. They also give the native fauna vital habitat and food supplies.

1.2. Ecological Advantages

- **Biodiversity:** By giving native insects, birds, and pollinators a place to live and eat, native plants contribute to the health of nearby ecosystems. This promotes a healthy, balanced atmosphere.

- **Soil Health:** Deep root systems of native plants improve soil structure, lessen erosion, and increase water infiltration. These features all contribute to the health of the soil.

- **Water Conservation:** Compared to non-native species, many native plants are drought-tolerant and use less water. As a result, less irrigation is required, which helps preserve water supplies.

1.3. Selecting Local Plants

- **Local Resources:** For advice on native plant species appropriate for your area, contact your local extension office, native plant societies, or gardening centres. They can offer guidance on choosing, taking care of, and maintaining plants.

- **Planting Points to Remember:** Select native plants that are compatible with the soil type, moisture content, and light conditions of your garden. To develop a garden that is resilient and diversified, include a variety of species.

1.4. Using Native Plants in Design

- **Habitat Creation:** Plan your garden such that it has a range of native plants with varying textures, heights, and colours. This produces a landscape that is both aesthetically pleasing and environmentally useful.

Plant native flowering plants in Pollinator Gardens to draw pollinators like hummingbirds, butterflies, and bees. Asters, coneflowers, and milkweed are a few examples.

2. Vertical Gardening: Adding Greenery and Making the Most of Space

2.1. An Overview of Vertical Gardening in

- **Definition:** Vertical gardening is the practice of cultivating plants on vertical surfaces, such as towers, trellises, or walls, or in vertically piled layers. It's a practical answer for tiny or urban gardens with constrained space.

- **Benefits:** Vertical gardening makes optimal use of available resources, such as water and sunshine, and maximises available space. It also improves visual attractiveness. It also offers chances to cultivate a large range of plants in constrained spaces.

2.2. Vertical Garden Types

- **Wall Planters:** To grow plants vertically on fences, walls or building exteriors, use wall-mounted planters, pockets or panels. Materials such as fabric, metal, or wood can be used to create these structures.

- **Trellises and Arbours:** To support climbing plants like peas, beans, and cucumbers, install trellises or arbours.

These buildings can be utilised to create shaded sections or garden dividers, and they also offer vertical appeal.

- Vertical Planter Towers: Grow herbs, flowers, or little veggies in tier-filled planter towers or stackable pots. These towers, which are suitable for patios, balconies, and little gardens, maximise available area.

2.3. Choosing Vegetables for Indoor Gardens

- Climbing Plants: For vertical constructions, use vining or climbing plants like hops, clematis, or morning gloryries. These plants can cover arbours or trellises because they naturally grow vertically.

- Compact Varieties: Select dwarf or compact plant types that work well in vertical containers. Smaller containers are ideal for flowering plants like petunias and succulents, as well as herbs like basil, parsley, and thyme.

2.4. Vertical Garden Design and Installation

- **Structural Support:** Make sure that the vertical supports are firmly in place and strong enough to hold the weight of the plants and growing medium. Make use of the right materials and anchors for the given wall or surface.

- **Maintenance and Watering:** Because of their exposure and little soil volume, vertical gardens frequently need more regular watering. To control water requirements, use effective irrigation systems like drip irrigation or self-watering pots.

- **Sunshine and Airflow:** Place vertical gardens where the plants will receive enough sunshine. To avoid mould and mildew, especially in vertical gardens with dense vegetation, make sure there is adequate airflow.

3. Blending Vertical and Native Plants

3.1 Integration's Advantages

- **Enhanced Biodiversity:** Using vertical gardening methods in conjunction with native plants produces a habitat that benefits nearby species and enhances the ecological value of your garden.

- **Efficient Use of Space:** You may make the most of your limited space while preserving ecological benefits by incorporating native plants into vertical gardens. This method works well for little residential spaces or urban gardens.

3.2. Useful Advice

- **Select Compatible Plants:** Go for natural plants, such as climbing or trailing types, that are appropriate for vertical gardening settings. Make sure the light and moisture levels in the vertical garden are just right for these plants.

- **Considerations for Design:** To build a dynamic and eye-catching vertical garden, incorporate native species with varying growth habits and flowering periods. Consider seasonal variations and upkeep requirements.

3.3. Native Vertical Plant Examples

- **Climbing Native Vines:** Cover trellises and arbours with native vines such as honeysuckle, wild grape, and Virginia creeper. These plants draw pollinators and produce lovely leaves.

- **Trailing Native Plants:** Use hanging baskets or vertical planters to plant trailing native plants, such as wild ginger or creeping thyme. These plants provide vertical areas more texture and foliage.

There are many ways to improve the sustainability, usefulness, and aesthetic appeal of your garden, including using native and vertical plants. Utilising native plants not only helps local ecosystems but also uses less resources; vertical gardening techniques allow you to maximise space and provide visual interest.

By incorporating these strategies into your garden design, you can produce a flourishing, environmentally responsible landscape that enhances your living area and the surrounding area. Accepting native and vertical plants can make your garden a more resilient, greener oasis, regardless of gardening ability level.

➢ Water-Efficient Gardening Advice: Effective Techniques for a thriving garden

A healthy and sustainable garden requires careful water management, particularly in regions that are vulnerable to drought or have limited water supplies. Using water-saving methods guarantees that your plants get the proper amount of moisture for healthy growth while also lessening the environmental impact of your garden. This guide offers doable advice and techniques for maintaining a lush, fruitful garden while preserving water.

1. Watering Methods That Work

1.1. Watering via Drip

- **Overview:** Using a system of emitters and tubing, drip irrigation supplies water straight to the root zone of the plant. This technique uses less water since it reduces runoff and evaporation.

- **Benefits:** By directing water just to the root zone, drip irrigation minimises water waste, suppresses weed growth, and is easily modified to suit the requirements of various plants.

- **Installation:** To target different plants, install a drip irrigation system with adjustable emitters. To guarantee constant hydration and automate watering schedules, use a timer.

1.2. Hoses for Soaking

- **Overview:** Water is gradually released from porous hoses along their length via soaker hoses. They are perfect for irrigating row crops and garden beds.

- **Benefits:** By putting water directly into the soil, soaker hoses minimise water waste, minimise evaporation, and distribute moisture evenly.

- **Implementation:** Bury soaker hoses beneath mulch or place them on the soil's surface. To regulate the length of the watering, connect them to a water supply and set a timer.

1.3. Watering by Hand

- **Overview:** Hand watering entails putting water directly on plants using a hose or watering can equipped with a spray nozzle.

- **Advantages:** Hand watering is beneficial for tiny gardens or plants in containers since it gives you exact control over how much water is applied.

- **Installation:** To minimise evaporation, water plants in the early morning or late at night. To prevent soil erosion, use a fine-spray watering can or soaker nozzle.

2. Methods for Mulching and Soil

2.1. Amendments to Soil

- **Organic Matter:** Adding organic matter, like aged manure or compost, strengthens the structure of the soil and increases its capacity to hold moisture.

- **Advantages:** Improved soil quality increases water retention, lessens the need for routine irrigation, and promotes strong plant development.

- **Implementation**: Before planting, incorporate organic matter into the soil; also, top-dress garden beds with compost on a regular basis.

2.2. The Practice of Mulching

- **Overview:** Mulching is the process of covering the soil surface surrounding plants with a layer of either organic or inorganic material.

- **Advantages:** Mulch controls soil temperature, discourages weed growth, helps keep soil moist, and lessens evaporation.

- **Implementation:** Surround plants and garden beds with a 2-4 inch layer of mulch, such as wood chips, straw, or leaves. To keep the coverage, replenish the mulch as necessary.

2.3. Monitoring Soil Moisture

- **Overview:** By revealing the soil's present water content, soil moisture monitoring helps avoid over- or under-watering.

- **Advantages:** Precise moisture monitoring guarantees that plants get the proper quantity of moisture and minimises water waste.

- **Implementation:** Examine the soil manually or with soil moisture meters. Water plants when the soil feels dry, about one to two inches down, and modify watering schedules according to moisture content.

3. Choosing and Placing Plants

3.1. Plants Resistant to Drought

- **Overview:** Plants that can withstand drought are adapted to require less water and can flourish in arid environments.

- **Advantages:** Selecting plants that can withstand drought lowers the requirement for regular watering and guarantees a more resilient garden.

- **Installation:** For your garden, choose drought-tolerant native plants such as decorative grasses, succulents, and lavender. Put plants together that require similar amounts of water.

3.2. Plant Classification

- Overview: Plants with comparable water requirements can be grouped together to decrease water waste and enable more effective watering.

- Advantages: Plant grouping helps to prevent overwatering of drought-tolerant species and guarantees that water is given where it is most needed.

- Implementation : Group plants that require a lot of moisture together and keep drought-tolerant kinds apart. Arrange plants according to their water requirements.

3.3. Adequate Alignment

- Overview: Proper plant spacing promotes improved air circulation and lessens fertiliser and water competition.

- Advantages: Optimal spacing reduces the chance of illness, enhances water absorption, and encourages robust plant development.

- **Implementation:** To guarantee that every plant has adequate access to water, adhere to the prescribed spacing standards for each species of plant and refrain from overcrowding.

4. Strategies for Conserving Water

4.1. Harvesting Rainwater

- **Overview:** Gathering and preserving rainwater for irrigation purposes is known as rainwater harvesting.

- **Benefits:** Harvesting rainwater decreases water expenses, lessens dependency on municipal sources, and gives plants natural, chemical-free water.

- **Implementation:** To collect rainwater from downspouts, install cisterns or rain barrels. Utilise rainwater collection for outdoor applications such as lawn watering.

4.2. Recycling Greywater

- **Overview:** Greywater recycling is the practice of repurposing wastewater from washing machines, sinks and showers for irrigation.

- **Advantages:** Reusing greywater promotes sustainable gardening techniques, lowers wastewater discharge, and conserves fresh water.

- **Implementation:** Redirect domestic water sources to garden irrigation by using a greywater collection system. Make sure that no dangerous chemicals or detergents are present in the greywater.

4.3. Effective Scheduling of Irrigation

- **Overview:** To reduce water waste, plants should be watered at the best times and frequencies through efficient irrigation scheduling.

- **Advantages:** When plants are scheduled appropriately, they receive enough moisture without using too much water, which lowers their total water use.

- **Installation:** To reduce evaporation, water plants in the early morning or late at night. Adapt watering schedules to the demands of the plants and the weather.

Using water-saving gardening methods encourages stronger, more resilient plants in addition to helping preserve important resources. You may develop a successful garden that meets your needs and the needs of the environment by applying conservation measures, implementing effective watering practices, enhancing the health of the soil, and choosing appropriate plants.

Water-efficient gardening is a useful and efficient approach to support sustainable living while reaping the rewards of a lush, fruitful garden. Take use of these techniques to improve your gardening methods and contribute positively to water saving initiatives.

Chapter 7

Mindful Consumption

In a world where technology is developing at a breakneck pace and consumerism is on the rise, the idea of conscious consumption has become essential to leading a more ethical and sustainable life. Making deliberate decisions about our purchases, resource usage, and the effects of our consuming habits on the environment and society are all part of mindful consumption. This manual examines the fundamentals of mindful consumption, as well as the advantages and doable tactics for bringing awareness into regular purchase decisions.

1. Having a Conscious Consumption

1.1. Concept and Guidelines

- **Definition**: Conscious consumption is the process of selecting goods and services with consideration and knowledge.

- **Fundamentals:** The three guiding concepts of mindful consumerism are accountability, intentionality, and awareness. This entails being aware of the resources consumed, comprehending the lifecycle of products, and thinking through the moral ramifications of the decisions we make.

1.2. The Influence of Customer Decisions

- **Environmental Impact:** Through waste production, pollution, and resource depletion, our consumption habits have a major negative impact on the environment. Minimising the ecological footprint and encouraging sustainable habits are two ways that mindful consumerism aims to lessen these effects.

- **Social Impact:** Decisions made by consumers have an impact on social conditions, such as community well-being and labour practices. Mindful consumerism aids in the advancement of social justice and enhances working conditions by endorsing ethical companies and fair trade practices.

2. Advantages of Consuming With Mind

2.1. Advantages for the Environment

- **Resource Conservation:** By encouraging the more economical use of resources, mindful consumption lowers waste and raw material consumption. This eases the burden on ecosystems and contributes to the conservation of natural resources.

- **Reduced Pollution:** People can lessen pollution and greenhouse gas emissions by choosing environmentally friendly products and cutting back on wasteful spending. This helps to make the land, water, and air cleaner.

2.2. Benefits to Society

- **Support for Ethical Practices:** Choosing goods from businesses that value moral standards like fair labour practices and community involvement is part of mindful consumerism. This enhances the standard of living for employees and supports ethical business operations.

- **Empowerment and Awareness:** Mindful consumption practices enable people to make better informed decisions and increase their awareness of the consequences of such decisions. This motivates constructive change and develops a sense of accountability.

2.3. Individual Advantages

- **Financial Savings:** Conscientious consumption frequently results in more deliberate purchases, which can cut down on impulsive purchases and save money over time. Spending can be decreased overall by making quality product investments and cutting waste.

- **Enhanced Well-Being:** People can feel more satisfied and have a feeling of purpose if their purchase patterns are in line with their environmental concerns and personal values. This enhances contentment and general well-being.

3. Mindful Consumption Strategies

3.1. Comparing Needs and Wants

- **Needs Assessment:** Determine whether an item is a luxury or a need before making a purchase. Set priorities for your most basic needs and refrain from making pointless purchases that lead to waste and overconsumption.

- **Mindful Reflection:** Examine why you desire a specific thing and whether it is consistent with your objectives and values. Steer clear of rash purchases and take your time making thoughtful decisions.

3.2. Examine and Select Eco-Friendly Products

- **Product Research:** Before making a purchase, find out how a product will affect society and the environment. Seek out labels and certifications that speak to sustainability, such those that say "organic," "fair trade," or "eco-friendly."

- **Higher Quality Than Quantity:** Choose long-lasting, robust items with superior quality. Purchasing high-quality products minimises waste and lessens the need for frequent replacements.

3.3. Assist Ethical Brands

- **Ethical Sourcing:** Give your support to businesses and brands who place a high value on moral standards including respect for the environment, fair labour practices, and responsible sourcing. Make sure brands fit your beliefs and ideals by doing some research on them.

- **Local and Small Businesses:** As opposed to giant corporations with international supply chains, local and small businesses tend to be more environmentally conscious and give back to the community.

3.4. Utilise, Recycle, and Reduce

- **Decrease Consumption:** Pay attention to lowering your total consumption by purchasing fewer single-use items and exercising caution while making purchases. Adopt minimalist living habits to cut down on clutter and simplify your life.

- **Reuse and Upcycle:** Apply the ideas of upcycling and reusing by giving objects a new lease on life. This increases product longevity and lessens waste.

- **Recycle Correctly:** Make sure recyclables are sorted and processed correctly according to recycling requirements. Steer clear of polluting recyclables and back programs that encourage efficient recycling techniques.

3.5. Make Eating Conscious

- **Sustainable Food Choices:** To lessen the environmental effect of food production and transportation, choose seasonal, organic, and locally sourced foods. Plan your meals and find inventive ways to use leftovers to reduce food waste.

- **Mindful Eating:** Make mindful eating a habit by enjoying meals, being aware of portion sizes, and putting aside distractions. This decreases food waste and encourages better eating practices.

4. Including Mindful Eating in Daily Life

4.1. Establish a Plan for Consumption

- **Set Goals:** Make sure you have well-defined objectives for cutting waste, endorsing ethical companies, and choosing sustainably. Keep an eye on your development and adapt as necessary.

- **Budgeting:** Set aside money in a way that reflects your priorities and ideals. Spending should be directed towards ethical and sustainable methods.

4.2. Instruct and Involve

- **Remain Informed**:** Continue to learn about ethical brands, sustainable methods, and environmental challenges. Keep up with the latest advancements and fashions in conscious consumption.

- **Collaborate with Others:** Talk to friends, family, and people in the community about what you know and have experienced. Talk about mindful consumption and inspire others to follow in your footsteps.

4.3. Take the Lead

- **Model Behaviour:** Set a good example for others by practicing mindful consumption yourself. Teach people to make thoughtful decisions and the advantages of implementing sustainable practices.

- **Advocate for Change:** Encourage and support laws and programs that advance moral behaviour and sustainability. Participate in movements and organisations that promote constructive social and environmental change.

Making decisions that are ethical, sustainable, and beneficial to the environment can be achieved through mindful consumption. Through the adoption of the values of responsibility, awareness, and intentionality, we can improve our general well-being, lessen our impact on the environment, and promote moral behaviour.

It takes careful consideration, reasoned judgement, and a dedication to constructive change to put mindful consuming practices into practice. We may design a more sustainable and satisfying lifestyle by carefully assessing our needs, endorsing sustainable goods and companies, and implementing waste-reduction strategies.

Mindful consumption provides a way to consume in a way that is more in tune with the environment and society as we work through the challenges of contemporary consumerism. We can help create a more sustainable future and encourage others to join us on this significant journey by making thoughtful decisions and setting a good example.

➢ Minimalism and Ethical Shopping

Minimalism and ethical buying have become popular complimentary behaviours in the pursuit of a more sustainable and meaningful living. These habits can greatly reduce our environmental impact and improve our quality of life. Both strategies place an emphasis on considerate consumption, choosing quality over quantity, and adhering to principles that promote both individual welfare and environmental sustainability. This manual examines the relationship between minimalism and ethical shopping and provides doable methods for incorporating these ideas into daily life.

1. Getting to Know Minimalism

1.1. Concept and Guidelines

- **Definition:** The idea of minimalism is a way of living that promotes intentionality and simplicity in one's actions and belongings. It emphasises cutting back on excess, setting priorities for what is really important, and getting rid of clutter.

- **Principles:** Decluttering, deliberate living, and emphasising experiences above material belongings are among the fundamental ideas of minimalism. The philosophy of minimalism urges people to reduce their consumption and create space for the things that truly enrich their lives.

1.2. The Advantages of Simplicity

- **Reduced Clutter:** A minimalist lifestyle helps get rid of mental and material clutter, making a home that is more orderly and tranquil.

- **Financial Savings:** Minimalism can result in significant financial savings and lower impulsive spending by emphasising necessities and eschewing pointless expenditures.

- **Enhanced Well-Being:** By prioritising quality over quantity and enabling people to make important experiences investments, minimalism fosters a sense of freedom and fulfilment.

2. Overview of Ethical Shopping

2.1. Concept and Guidelines

- **Definition:** Ethical shopping is the process of choosing products based on moral principles including justice, sustainability of the environment, and social responsibility. It aims to promote goods and companies that benefit both people and the environment.

- **Principles:** Choosing eco-friendly products, avoiding brands with unethical methods, and supporting fair trade are important ethical buying behaviours. Transparency, integrity, and the welfare of the environment and labourers are prioritised in ethical buying.

2.2. Advantages of Ethical Purchasing

- **Beneficial Impact:** Ethical purchasing promotes companies that value moral standards, such as decent working conditions and environmentally friendly production techniques, which benefits society and the environment.

- **Informed Choices:** Customers can stimulate demand for ethical products and persuade businesses to adopt more conscientious methods by making educated purchase decisions.

- **Personal Fulfilment:** When consumers make ethical purchase selections, their values are matched, which increases their sense of purpose and fulfilment.

3. Combining Ethical Buying with Minimalism

3.1. Prioritise and Simplify

- **Identify Needs:** Prioritising and recognising true needs is the first step towards minimalism. Consider whether the item is necessary and how it fits with your values before making a purchase.

- **Quality Above Quantity:** Place more emphasis on a product's lifetime and quality than its quantity. Select well-made products with timeless appeal and longevity.

3.2. Make Knowledgeable Choices

- **Research Brands:** Before making a purchase, look into a company's or brand's ethical policies. Seek out certifications like cruelty-free, organic, or Fair Trade labels.

- **Transparency and Accountability:** Give your support to companies who are open and honest about their labour methods, environmental effect, and supplier chain. Steer clear of businesses that use dubious or unethical techniques.

3.3. Encourage Ethical and Sustainable Products

- **Eco-Friendly Materials:** Choose goods manufactured from recycled or sustainable materials. Steer clear of single-use plastics and choose for products with the least amount of environmental impact.

- **Fair Trade and Ethical Labour:** Buy goods from businesses that value ethical labour standards, such as paying workers a fair salary and providing safe working conditions. Encourage small companies and craftspeople who boost the regional economy

3.4. Make Conscious Consumption Practices

- **Mindful Purchasing:** Go about your buying mindfully and with a goal. Steer clear of impulsive purchases and think through each one's long-term effects.

- **Reduce Waste:** Put waste-reduction strategies into action by fixing broken objects rather than throwing them away and recycling or donating anything you no longer need.

3.5. Adopt A Minimalist Lifestyle

- **Declutter Often:** Examine your possessions on a regular basis and get rid of everything that isn't needed. Things that are still in good condition can be recycled or donated.

- **Simplify Spaces:** Focus on the necessities and get rid of extras to create a minimalist living space. Organise your area to make it more functional and less cluttered.

4. Useful Advice for Conscientious Minimalism and Ethical Buying

4.1. Make a list of things to buy

- **Plan Ahead:** To prevent impulsive purchases and maintain focus on your needs, make a list of necessary products before you go shopping.

- **Determine Priorities:** Sort objects according to quality and necessity. Adhere to your shopping list to reduce pointless purchases.

4.2. Select Vintage and Second-Hand Items

- **Second-Hand Shops:** Look for pre-owned things in thrift stores, secondhand shops, and internet marketplaces. This lessens waste and promotes a circular economy.

- **Vintage Finds:** Look for upcycled or vintage goods with a distinct character and longevity. Antique goods frequently have less of an influence on the environment.

4.3. Encourage Small and Local Businesses

- **Local Artists:** Help out your neighborhood's handicrafters and artisans who use ethical sources to create their handcrafted goods. This lessens the transport sector's carbon footprint and supports local economies.

- **Farmers' Markets:** Purchase locally produced, fresh produce and goods at farmers' markets. This lessens the negative effects of food transportation on the environment and promotes sustainable agriculture.

4.4. Educate Others as Well as Yourself

- **Remain Informed:** Continually acquaint yourself with the consequences of your consumption decisions and ethical shopping techniques. Keep abreast of emerging ethical brands and trends in sustainability.

- **Exchange Information:** Encourage ethical buying and mindful simplicity in your neighbourhood. Disseminate facts and inspire others to follow suit.

A powerful combination of ideals that support a more sustainable, fulfilling, and responsible lifestyle is represented by minimalism and ethical buying. Adopting a minimalist lifestyle allows people to focus on what really matters, declutter, and simplify their lives. In the meanwhile, shopping ethically guarantees that our decisions about consumption reflect our values and have a good impact on the environment and society.

Intentionality, awareness, and a dedication to making wise judgements are necessary for incorporating these ideas into daily living. We may achieve a harmonious balance between our wants and the health of the world by practicing mindful consumerism. We improve our own quality of life and help create a more fair and equitable society by endorsing ethical and sustainable behaviours.

Adopting a minimalist lifestyle and ethical shopping practices can help us manage the complexity of contemporary consumerism and pave the way for a more sustainable future and increased fulfilment. We may encourage positive change and contribute to a world that is healthier and more equal by making thoughtful decisions and setting an example.

➢ Benefits of Buying Second-Hand

Purchasing used goods has grown in popularity as more people become aware of its advantages for their own and the environment's well-being. By lowering waste and saving resources, secondhand buying helps sustainability initiatives in addition to offering financial benefits. This book examines the many advantages of buying used goods and explains why doing so is a wise financial and environmental decision.

1. Environmental Advantages

1.1. Waste Reduction

- Reducing Landfill Contributions: Buying used goods helps keep goods out of landfills. Reusing pre-existing objects helps to cut down on the amount of waste that ends up in landfills, which reduces pollution to the environment and saves landfill space.

- Extending Product Life: Buying used goods prolongs their lifespan and keeps them from going bad too soon. This method encourages the circular economy, in which goods are recycled, repaired, and reused as opposed to being thrown away.

1.2. Resource Conservation

- Reducing Demand for New Resources: Purchasing used goods lowers the demand for new goods, which in turn lowers the amount of energy and raw resources needed for manufacturing. This lessens the negative effects of production operations on the environment and contributes to the conservation of natural resources.

- **Reducing Carbon Footprint:** A major portion of greenhouse gas emissions are caused by the shipping and manufacturing of new goods. Selecting used goods might help you reduce your carbon footprint because they usually have less of an impact on the environment than newly made things.

2. Financial Gains

2.1. Savings on Costs

- **Affordable Prices:** Compared to new products, used goods are frequently far less expensive. This makes it possible for you to get premium goods for a much lower price, which adds up to significant savings over time.

- **Value for Money:** A lot of lightly used, still-excellent second-hand goods provide exceptional value for the money. For a lot less money, you can find things that are just as good as new.

2.2. Unusual Discovery

- **Distinctive and Vintage things:** Unique, vintage, or one-of-a-kind things that are not carried by chain retailers are frequently found through second-hand shopping. This enables you to locate unique items that give your house or clothing personality.

- **Hidden Treasures:** You can find unusual or discontinued things in thrift stores and second-hand shops like a treasure. Investigating these shops may reveal priceless or unusual items that you would not find in traditional retail environments.

3. Advantages for Society

3.1. Assisting Neighbourhoods

- **Local Businesses:** Since many thrift stores are run by people in the area, your purchases will directly benefit small companies and regional economies. Both job creation and community development may benefit from this.

- **Charitable Organisations:** A lot of thrift stores are operated by non-profits or charitable organisations. Purchasing from these retailers advances their goals and helps fund social services, community initiatives, and other charity endeavours.

3.2. Encouraging Ecological Lifestyles

- **Raising knowledge:** Purchasing used goods contributes to increasing public knowledge of the advantages of sustainable living and mindful consumption. Your decisions have the power to affect other people and advance a larger movement for environmental stewardship.

- **Educational chances:** Purchasing used goods can offer educational chances to learn about the negative effects of consumerism on the environment and the significance of waste reduction.

4. Practical and High-Quality Advantages

4.1. Security of the Quality

- Well-Made Products: A lot of used goods are sturdy and well-made. Certain modern, mass-produced products can't compare to the high-quality materials and skill used in the construction of older products, particularly furniture and appliances.

- Tested Durability: Used and tested over time, second-hand items can provide insight into their dependability and longevity. When making a purchase, this useful feature might provide you peace of mind.

4.2. Customisation Possibility

- DIY Projects: Purchasing used goods gives you the opportunity to adapt and repurpose them to fit your needs and unique taste. With inventive DIY ideas, you may turn used furniture, clothes, and other items into something totally unique.

- **Restoration and Repair:** Buying used goods enables you to take on rewarding and reasonably priced restoration or repair jobs. This lends credence to the idea of prolonging product lifetimes via upkeep and handling.

5. Buying Advice on Used Items

5.1. Purchase Knowledge

- **Charity Shops and Thrift Stores:** These establishments sell a variety of used products, such as furniture, clothing, and household items. They are frequently a useful place to start looking for reasonably priced and distinctive goods.

- **Online Marketplaces:** You may find a wide range of used goods, from electronics to vintage treasures, on websites and applications like eBay, Facebook Marketplace, and Craigslist. They provide ease of use and the chance to locate particular products.

5.2. Examine Prior to Buying

- **Check Condition:** Carefully examine used goods for indications of wear, damage, or faults. Before making a purchase, make sure the item fits your quality criteria and is in good functioning order.

- **Verify Authenticity:** To prevent buying fake or misrepresented goods, confirm the provenance and authenticity of precious or collectible objects.

5.3. Bargain and Contrast

- **Bargain:** A lot of consignment shops and vendors are amenable to haggling. If you are purchasing many goods, don't be afraid to ask for discounts or to make a reasonable offer.

- **Compare Options:** To get the greatest offers and make sure you are getting the best value for your money, compare comparable items across various retailers or online platforms.

Purchasing used goods is a wise and sustainable decision that has several advantages, including preserving the environment, saving money, helping out the community, and finding one-of-a-kind finds. Adopting second-hand shopping behaviours can help create a circular economy, cut waste, and encourage moral consumerism.

Keep in mind that every purchase you make as you venture into the world of second-hand shopping helps you live a more responsible and sustainable lifestyle. Secondhand shopping provides a multitude of chances to make thoughtful decisions that are in line with your values and promote a healthier world, whether you are looking for reasonably priced necessities, unique finds or inspiration for creative endeavours.

Chapter 8

Renewable Energy: Energising the Future for Sustainability

Renewable energy has become essential for sustaining a sustainable future as the globe struggles with the effects of climate change and the depletion of non-renewable resources. Renewable energy sources may supply a sizable amount of the world's energy demands and are plentiful, eco-friendly, and replace fossil fuels. This guide examines the several types of renewable energy, their advantages, and the opportunities and problems that come with implementing them.

1. Renewable Energy Types

1.1. Energy from Sunlight

- **Description:** Solar energy uses the sun's beams to generate heat or electricity. Solar thermal systems, which use sunlight to heat fluids, or photovoltaic (PV) cells, which turn sunlight directly into energy, can do this.

- **Advantages:** Solar energy is generally accessible and abundant. It lessens reliance on fossil fuels and greenhouse gas emissions. From tiny residential systems to massive solar farms, solar installations can be adjusted to fulfil a variety of purposes.

- **Difficulties:** Weather and geographic location affect how effective solar energy is. Despite a considerable upfront cost and space requirement, solar panel prices have been declining over time.

1.2. Energy from Wind

- **Description:** Wind turbines are used to harness the kinetic energy of the wind to produce power. Usually, wind farms—either onshore or offshore—install these turbines.

- **Benefits:** Wind energy emits no greenhouse gases while in use, making it a clean and renewable resource. Once deployed, it can be used in many places, including remote ones, and has comparatively minimal operational costs.

- **Difficulties:** Depending on the wind conditions, wind energy generation may be sporadic. Concerns have also been raised on how wind turbines may affect nearby people and wildlife.

1.3. The use of hydropower

- **Description:** Using the flow of water from dams or rivers to move turbines, hydropower, also known as hydroelectric power, produces electricity. It is among the most traditional and extensively utilised kind of sustainable energy.

- **Advantages:** Hydropower offers a steady and dependable energy supply. It's a flexible resource for supply and demand management since it can store energy in reservoirs and release it when needed.

- Difficulties: Large-scale dam construction can have detrimental effects on the environment and society, uprooting communities and destroying habitat. Concerns exist over how the environment may affect river ecosystems.

1.4. Energy from Biomass

- Description: Organic materials like plant and animal waste are used to produce biomass energy. These materials can be directly utilised to produce heat and power, or they can be processed into biofuels like ethanol and biodiesel.

- Benefits: By utilising resources that may otherwise degrade in landfills, biomass energy helps reduce waste. It can also support the economic development of rural areas and offer a dependable and controlled energy supply.

- **Difficulties:** If biomass energy generation is not handled responsibly, it may compete with food production and result in deforestation. Although emissions from it are typically less than those from fossil fuels, they might nevertheless occur.

1.5. Energy from the Earth

- **Description:** The heat that is retained beneath the surface of the Earth is the source of geothermal energy. Heat pumps and geothermal power plants can be used to directly heat buildings or produce electricity from this heat.

- **Benefits:** With a minimal land footprint, geothermal energy is a dependable and steady power source. Regardless of the weather, it can consistently deliver energy with little greenhouse gas emissions.

- **Difficulties:** The development of geothermal energy can be costly and location-specific. Drilling below the surface and the possibility of induced seismicity (earthquakes) are other dangers.

2. Advantages of Green Energy

2.1. Advantages for the Environment

- Reduction in Greenhouse Gas Emissions: When operating, renewable energy sources emit little to no greenhouse gases, which contributes to reducing air pollution and mitigating climate change.

- Preservation of Natural Resources: Renewable energy sources do not deplete finite resources because they are naturally regenerated, in contrast to fossil fuels. By doing this, natural habitats and ecosystems are preserved.

2.2. Financial Gains

- Job Creation: Manufacturing, installation, maintenance, and research & development are among the job categories where the renewable energy industry creates jobs. It might boost regional economies and generate a sizable number of new employment.

Energy Independence: By putting money into renewable energy, nations can lessen their need on imported fossil fuels, improving stability and security in the energy sector. Additionally, this helps protect economies from erratic international energy markets.

2.3 Health Advantages

- **Improved Air Quality:** Since renewable energy sources emit fewer pollutants into the atmosphere than fossil fuels do, the air is cleaner and the risks of respiratory and cardiovascular illnesses linked to air pollution are lower.

- **Reduced Environmental Impact:** The extraction and burning of fossil fuels causes less environmental harm than cleaner energy sources, which benefits communities and ecosystems.

3. Problems and Their Fixes

3.1. Dependability and Intermittency

- **Difficulty:** A lot of renewable energy sources, like wind and solar power, are sporadic and weather-dependent. This may make it more difficult to keep up a steady source of energy.

- **Remedy:** Supply and demand can be more evenly distributed by putting energy storage devices—like batteries and pumped hydro storage—into place. Reliability can also be increased by upgrading grid infrastructure and combining several renewable energy sources.

3.2. Expenses and Investment at First

- **Difficulty:** The initial costs of renewable energy systems, including those related to installation, research, and development, can be substantial.

- **Remedy:** Renewable energy system costs are declining as economies of scale are reached and technology progresses. Lowering the cost barriers to adoption can also be accomplished with the aid of government subsidies, financing choices, and incentives.

3.3. Environmental Impact and Land Use

- **Challenge:** Some renewable energy projects, such massive wind and solar farms, need a lot of land and may have an adverse effect on the surrounding ecosystems and species.

- **Remedy:** The effects on the environment can be reduced with careful site selection and planning. Technological advancements like offshore wind turbines and vertical farming can also lessen the disturbance of the environment and the utilisation of land.

3.4. Integration and Development of Technology

- **Challenge:** To assure efficiency and compatibility, the integration of renewable energy into current energy systems necessitates breakthroughs in infrastructure and technology.

- **Remedy:** Successful integration requires ongoing research and development in the fields of energy storage, smart grids, and renewable energy technology. Governments, businesses, and academics working together can spur innovation and advancement.

4. Renewable Energy's Future

Renewable energy has a bright future because of ongoing technological developments and a growing global commitment to sustainability. Renewable energy sources will contribute more and more to the world's energy mix as they become more economical and efficient.

4.1. Innovations in Technology

- **Advanced Energy Storage:** The flexibility and dependability of renewable energy systems will be improved by advancements in energy storage technology, such as thermal storage solutions and next-generation batteries.

- **Smart Grids:** As smart grid technologies advance, renewable energy management and distribution will be enhanced, allowing for more effective integration and use of various energy sources.

4.2. International Programs and Regulations

- **Climate Agreements:** Investment and adoption will be fuelled by international accords and domestic laws designed to lower greenhouse gas emissions and promote renewable energy.

- **Incentives and Support:** The industry will expand and the shift to renewable energy will happen more quickly if subsidies, tax breaks, and research funding are maintained.

4.3. Adoption and Public Awareness

- **Education and Advocacy:** Encouraging broad acceptance and support will come from educating the public about the advantages of renewable energy sources and promoting sustainable lifestyles.

- **Community Involvement:** Getting locals involved in renewable energy initiatives, including neighbourhood wind farms and solar cooperatives, can promote a sense of engagement and ownership.

A sustainable and resilient future depends heavily on renewable energy. We can lessen our dependency on fossil fuels, slow down climate change, and improve the environment by making use of natural resources including sunlight, wind, water, biomass, and geothermal heat.

A better energy landscape is being paved by continued technology developments, supportive laws, and growing public awareness, notwithstanding the hurdles inherent with renewable energy. We are getting closer to a sustainable future where everyone has access to abundant, dependable, and clean energy as long as we keep supporting and investing in renewable energy.

➢ Solar Panels and Wind Turbines: Utilising the Power of Nature

In the field of renewable energy, solar and wind power are two of the most well-known and quickly developing technologies. Both are essential to the shift away from fossil fuels and towards greener energy sources, providing long-term options for supplying our communities, businesses, and households with electricity. This article examines the operation of solar panels and wind turbines, as well as the advantages and disadvantages of using them.

1. Photovoltaic Cells

1.1. Solar Panel Operation

- **Photovoltaic Cells:** Photovoltaic (PV) panels, often known as solar panels, use semiconductor-based photovoltaic cells, such as silicon, to directly convert sunlight into electricity. These cells produce an electric current when sunlight strikes them because it excites the electrons.

- **Panel Composition:** Generally, a solar panel is made up of many PV cells that are linked in series and housed in a protective shell. Typically, solar panels are mounted on rooftops or in open spaces to maximise their exposure to sunlight.

- **Inverters:** These devices transform the direct current (DC) electricity produced by the panels into alternating current (AC), which is used in residences and commercial buildings. To guarantee effective utilisation, inverters also control the flow of electricity.

1.2. Solar Panel Advantages

- **Renewable and Abundant:** Wherever the sun shines, solar energy is a nearly infinite resource. Because of this, solar energy is a very renewable resource.

- **Reduces Electricity Bills:** You may lessen your dependency on the grid and cut down on your energy costs by producing your own electricity. It is frequently possible to sell created excess energy back to the grid, resulting in further financial gains.

- **Low Environmental Impact:** Compared to fossil fuel energy sources, solar panels produce no greenhouse gases while in operation and have a negligible environmental impact.

1.3. Solar Panel Difficulties

- **Intermittency:** The generation of solar energy is reliant on sunshine, which varies depending on the season and weather. To guarantee a steady supply, this intermittency necessitates solutions like energy storage or grid integration.

- **Initial Costs:** Although prices have been dropping, installing and buying solar panels can involve significant upfront costs. Rebates and financial incentives may help defray these expenses.

- **Space Requirements:** Installing solar panels requires a sufficient amount of space, which could be a problem in cities with small rooftops or shadow problems.

2. Generators of Wind

2.1. Functions of Wind Turbines

- **Wind Energy Conversion:** Wind turbines use mechanical energy to create electricity by converting the kinetic energy of the wind. The turbine's blades are turned by the wind, and this rotation spins a generator-connected rotor.

- **Turbine Components:** The rotor blades, hub, nacelle (which contains the generator and gearbox), and tower are the main parts of a wind turbine. To harness the most wind energy possible, the tower's height and the blades' layout have been optimised.

- **Grid Integration:** Using an inverter, the mechanical energy generated by the turbine is transformed into electrical energy and sent into the grid in a manner akin to that of solar panels.

2.2. Advantages of Wind Generators

- **Clean and Renewable:** There are no greenhouse gas emissions or air pollutants from wind energy, making it a clean energy source. As long as the wind blows, it is a renewable resource that can be used.

- **Efficient Use of Space:** Wind farms can be situated onshore or offshore, and the area surrounding them is frequently suitable for grazing or other uses.

- **Economic Growth:** Manufacturing, installation, maintenance, and support services jobs are generated by the wind energy industry. Additionally, it boosts regional economies by making investments and building infrastructure.

2.3. Wind Turbine Difficulties

- **Intermittency and Variability:** Depending on wind speed and meteorological conditions, wind energy output can vary. This can be lessened by combining wind power with other renewable energy sources or by using energy storage technologies.

- **Visual and Noise Impact:** Wind turbines can produce noise and be aesthetically bothersome, which may worry the neighbours. These problems can be addressed with the help of improved technology and site selection.

- **Impact on Wildlife:** If wind turbines are not erected and designed appropriately, they may endanger birds and bats. Monitoring and careful planning can help reduce these effects.

3. Integrating Wind Turbines and Solar Panels

3.1. System Complementaries

- **Diversified Energy Supply:** A more dependable and steady energy source can be produced by combining wind turbines and solar panels. While wind energy can be more common at night or during certain seasons, solar energy is normally stronger during the day.

- **Optimised Performance:** You can balance out the individual intermittencies of both technologies and raise total energy production by merging them. Additionally, this strategy makes greater use of the resources that are accessible.

3.2. System Hybrids

- Integrated Solutions: Hybrid systems that incorporate energy storage devices, such batteries, along with solar and wind power can provide a more consistent and dependable energy source. These systems have the capacity to retain extra energy produced during periods of high production for use during times of low generation.

- Cost and Efficiency: Although hybrid systems may initially cost more, they are more dependable and efficient, which makes them appropriate for off-grid uses and distant areas.

4. Prospective Paths

4.1. Developments in Technology

- Improved Efficiency: Research and development efforts are continuously directed towards enhancing the effectiveness of wind turbines and solar panels. Technological developments in materials, design, and production are contributing to lower costs and higher energy output.

- Energy Storage Innovations: To solve the intermittent problems with solar and wind power, advances in energy storage technology, such as thermal storage systems and improved batteries, are crucial.

4.2. Investment and Policy

- Supportive Policies: The adoption of renewable energy technology is greatly aided by government incentives and policies. Supportive policies that can hasten the adoption of solar and wind energy include tax incentives, subsidies, and renewable energy standards.

- Investment and Research: The advancement of renewable energy technologies and their integration into current energy systems will depend on sustained investment in research and development as well as infrastructural upgrades.

4.3. International Cooperation

- **International Cooperation:** International cooperation is necessary to combat climate change and make the switch to renewable energy. The global adoption of solar and wind power can be accelerated by exchanging best practices, technologies, and expertise.

The participation of communities in renewable energy projects and decision-making procedures has the potential to improve acceptance and support of these technologies. Engaging the community locally can also result in more sustainable and efficient energy solutions.

Leading the charge in the renewable energy revolution are solar panels and wind turbines, which provide effective answers to the problems of resource depletion and climate change. Both technologies offer sustainable, clean energy that can cut greenhouse gas emissions dramatically and improve the health of the world.

Even though solar and wind energy have drawbacks, such as erratic output, high initial prices, and negative environmental effects, continued technological developments, encouraging regulations, and international cooperation are opening the door to a more sustainable energy future. We can transition to a more robust and sustainable energy system that benefits the environment and people by utilising the power of the sun and wind.

➢ Geothermal Heat and Cooling: Using the Natural Energy of the Earth

Geothermal heating and cooling systems make use of the heat that naturally exists on Earth to give homes and businesses effective, long-lasting temperature management. By utilising the steady temperatures found beneath, this technology provides an environmentally beneficial substitute for conventional heating and cooling systems by controlling indoor climates. This tutorial examines the advantages of geothermal systems as well as the drawbacks of using them.

1. Functions of Geothermal Systems

1.1. Foundational Ideas

- Earth's Natural Heat: The temperature of the Earth's crust stays largely constant all year long. Geothermal systems use this steady temperature as a source of heat and cold. Geothermal systems work independent of seasonal variations since the temperature gets more constant the deeper you go underground.

- Heat Exchange: Ground loops, a network of pipes buried in the ground or immersed in water, are used in geothermal systems. Through these pipes, a heat pump circulates a liquid—typically water or antifreeze—to transfer heat between the structure and the Earth. The system draws heat from the earth and moves it into the building throughout the winter. During the summer, the system works in the opposite direction, taking heat out of the building and releasing it into the earth.

1.2. Geothermal System Components

- Ground Loop: A ground loop is a system of pipes that are either buried beneath the surface of the earth or immersed in water. It can be erected in deep boreholes as a vertical loop, dispersed horizontally in trenches, or as a pond/lake loop in water bodies. Heat is exchanged between the earth and the loop.

- Heat Pump: Housed inside the structure, the heat pump serves as the system's central component. Its compressor and heat exchanger help to transmit heat from the ground loop to the air inside the building. The heat pump modifies the air's temperature according to the demands of the season.

- Distribution System: For forced air systems, the distribution system may consist of ductwork; for radiant floor heating, it may consist of a hydronic system. It distributes warm water or conditioned air throughout the structure.

2. Geothermal Heating and Cooling Advantages

2.1. Benefits for the Environment

- Reduced Greenhouse Gas Emissions: Compared to traditional heating and cooling systems that use fossil fuels, geothermal systems emit the fewest greenhouse gases. Both air quality and climate change mitigation are aided by this lowering.

- Sustainable Energy Source: Geothermal energy is sustainable and renewable since it draws from the ever-renewing interior heat of the Earth. It leaves little environmental trace and doesn't deplete natural resources.

2.2. Financial Gains

- **Lower Operating Costs:** Geothermal systems can be more expensive to build initially than conventional systems, but over time, they can save a significant amount of money. Compared to conventional systems, geothermal systems have the potential to save energy bills by 30% to 60%. They are extremely efficient.

- **Incentives and Rebates:** Financial incentives, tax credits, and rebates are provided by numerous governments and utilities in exchange for the installation of geothermal systems. These subsidies may be able to reduce the upfront expenses and lower the cost of geothermal systems.

2.3. Convenience and Effectiveness

- **Equal Temperature Control:** Geothermal systems eliminate hot and cold patches that are frequently encountered with conventional systems by providing equal and consistent heating and cooling. All year round, they keep the interior climate agreeable.

- **Silent Operation:** Because the ground loop is buried and the heat pump is housed inside the structure, geothermal systems are renowned for their silent operation, which reduces noise and disturbance.

3. Geothermal Heating and Cooling Challenges

3.1. High Start-Up Expenses

- **Installation Expenses:** The main drawback of geothermal systems is their high initial cost, which involves installing the heat pump and digging a trench for the ground loop. Adoption may be hampered by the expense, but this is frequently made up for by long-term benefits and incentives.

- **Site-Specific Factors:** Depending on the size of the property, the type of ground loop that is needed, and the state of the soil, there may be differences in the installation cost. To find the most economical solution, a thorough site study and planning are necessary.

3.2. Space and Installation Needs

- Space for Ground Loop: In heavily populated or metropolitan regions, space may be limited for the installation of a horizontal ground loop, which calls for a sizable amount of land. Although they are viable options, vertical loops and pond/lake loops might still need a significant amount of room and excavation.

- Expert Installation: Correct installation of geothermal systems necessitates certain training and experience. Collaborating with proficient experts is important to guarantee accurate installation and optimal system performance.

3.3. Sustaining and Extended Life

- Maintenance Requirements: Although geothermal systems often require less upkeep than conventional systems, they nevertheless require yearly servicing and inspections. To guarantee peak performance, the heat pump and ground loop should be inspected on a regular basis.

- **Component Lifespan:** The heat pump normally lasts 15 to 25 years, but the ground loop has a lengthy lifespan of 50 years or more. The system's lifespan can be increased and dependable functioning can be ensured with routine maintenance and prompt repairs.

4. Geothermal Technology Advances and Innovations

4.1. Designing an Enhanced System

- **Improved Heat Pumps:** New developments in heat pump science have produced units that are more dependable and efficient. Geothermal system performance is being improved by advances in compressor design, heat exchanger technology, and control systems.

- **Hybrid Systems:** In hybrid geothermal systems, solar panels and other renewable energy sources are combined with geothermal heating and cooling. These solutions boost overall efficiency and optimise energy use.

4.2. Recovery of Geothermal Heat

- Waste Heat Utilisation: To collect and repurpose extra heat from industrial processes or other sources, geothermal systems can be combined with waste heat recovery systems. This strategy can lower overall energy usage and increase energy efficiency.

4.3. Research and Adoption Worldwide

- International Growth: As more nations come to understand the advantages of sustainable energy, geothermal heating and cooling is becoming more and more commonplace. The performance of geothermal systems is being enhanced and their applications are being expanded through ongoing research and development.

- **Innovative Applications:** Scientists are investigating novel uses for geothermal energy, such as industrial operations and district heating systems for cities. These developments are helping geothermal technology become more widely used.

An effective and environmentally friendly way to control indoor temperature is through the use of geothermal heating and cooling systems. Geothermal systems provide substantial financial and environmental advantages by utilising the Earth's natural heat source. These advantages include less greenhouse gas emissions, lower energy costs, and reliable comfort.

Geothermal systems are becoming more widely available and effective despite the difficulties related to installation costs and space requirements, thanks to technological advancements and increasing global usage. In order to lessen our dependency on fossil fuels and to promote clean, renewable energy, geothermal heating and cooling will be essential as we look for ways to create a sustainable future.

Businesses and homes may make a long-term positive impact on the environment and reap the benefits of dependable and efficient temperature management by investing in geothermal technology.

Chapter 9

Green Home Design: Developing Eco-Friendly and Effective Living Environments

The goal of green home design, sometimes referred to as sustainable or eco-friendly home design, is to create homes that have as little of an impact on the environment as possible while maximising resource conservation, energy efficiency, and overall sustainability. Green house design is crucial for lowering our carbon footprint and fostering healthier living spaces as worries about climate change and resource depletion increase. This tutorial examines the fundamentals of green home design, important implementation techniques, and the advantages and difficulties of creating sustainable living environments.

1. Green Home Design Principles

1.1. Effectiveness of Energy Use

- **Optimising Energy Use:** Energy-efficient appliances, lighting, heating, and cooling systems are used in green home designs as a priority. Homeowners can minimise their carbon footprint and electricity costs by cutting back on their energy use.

- **Passive Solar Design:** This type of architecture arranges and plans a house to maximise the use of solar radiation for both heating and cooling. This entails employing thermal mass materials, putting windows in strategic locations, and adding overhangs to regulate shade and sun gain.

1.2. Preservation of Resources

- **Sustainable Materials:** An important part of designing a green home is using renewable and sustainable building materials. This involves the use of long-lasting, recyclable, and ethically sourced products with minimal negative effects on the environment.

- **Water Conservation:** Low-flow fixtures, rainwater harvesting systems, and drought-tolerant landscaping are examples of water-saving features found in green homes. Water expenses can be decreased and valuable resources can be preserved with efficient water use.

1.3. Quality of Indoor Environment

- **Healthy Indoor Air:** Using low-VOC paints and finishes, adding enough ventilation, and using materials that don't off-gas dangerous chemicals are all ways that greenhouse design aims to improve indoor air quality. As a result, residents live in a healthier atmosphere.

- **Natural Lighting and Ventilation:** Optimising natural light and ventilation can help to improve the comfort and well-being of the home's occupants by reducing the demand for artificial lighting and mechanical ventilation.

2. Crucial Approaches to Green House Design

2.1. Choosing and Orienting the Site

- **Choosing the Right Location:** A home's sustainability can be improved by choosing a place with ideal environmental conditions. To minimise energy use and transportation needs, factors including climate, geography, and closeness to amenities should be taken into account.

- **Optimal Orientation:** A house's orientation can enhance its energy efficiency by maximising its exposure to prevailing winds and natural light. Windows facing southwards receive more light, and summertime warmth can be avoided with appropriate shade.

2.2. Materials for Sustainable Construction

- **Recycled and Reclaimed Materials:** Utilising repurposed or recycled materials lessens waste and the need for new resources. Reclaimed wood, recycled metal, and rescued bricks are a few examples.

- **Fast Renewable Materials:** Sustainable substitutes for conventional building materials include bamboo, cork, and fast renewable fibres. They may be collected with little harm to the environment and grow swiftly.

2.3. Systems That Use Less Energy

- **High-Performance Insulation:** Energy consumption can be decreased and comfortable indoor temperatures can be maintained with proper insulation. High-performance insulating materials like fibreglass, cellulose, or spray foam are used in green homes.

- **Energy-Efficient HVAC Systems:** To reduce energy consumption, HVAC (heating, ventilation, and air conditioning) systems should be energy-efficient. Alternatives include variable speed motor air conditioners, high-efficiency furnaces, and geothermal heat pumps.

2.4. Handling of Water

- **Efficient Fixtures and Appliances:** Energy-efficient dishwashers and washing machines, as well as low-flow toilets, showerheads, and faucets, all contribute to water conservation and lower energy use.

- Rainwater Harvesting: Reducing water usage and relieving pressure on municipal water supplies can be accomplished by gathering and storing rainwater for drinking, toilet flushing, and irrigation.

2.5. Outdoor Spaces and Landscaping

- Drought-Tolerant Landscaping: Less irrigation and upkeep is required when native and drought-tolerant plants are used. Water conservation can be increased by implementing xeriscaping strategies like mulching and reducing the amount of turf.

- Green Roofs and Walls: Adding living walls and green roofs to urban areas can increase green space, lower stormwater runoff, and improve insulation.

3. Green Home Design's Advantages

3.1. The Effect on the Environment

- **Reduced Carbon Footprint:** By utilising sustainable materials and energy-efficient technologies, green homes help to reduce greenhouse gas emissions. This lessens the total impact on the environment and mitigates climate change.

- **Resource Conservation:** Green homes encourage responsible consumption and contribute to the preservation of natural resources by using sustainable building materials and effective water and energy systems.

3.2. Benefits to the Economy

- **Lower Utility Costs:** Because energy and water are used less in energy-efficient homes, utility costs are lower. The initial expenses of designing a green home can be compensated for by the savings from energy-efficient appliances and systems.

- **Increased Property Value:** Because of its sustainable features, lower operating expenses, and energy efficiency, green homes sometimes fetch a higher price when they are put up for sale. For homeowners wishing to sell their home, this can be a big benefit.

3.3. Comfort and Well-Being

- **Improved Indoor Air Quality:** Low-VOC materials and adequate ventilation create a better indoor atmosphere in green homes, which lowers the risk of allergies and respiratory problems.

- **Enhanced Comfort:** Passive solar heating and natural ventilation, two sustainable design elements, help create a more comfortable living space with consistent temperatures and high-quality air.

4. Green Home Design Difficulties

4.1. Initial Expenses

- **Initial Investment:** Compared to conventional building techniques, incorporating green design elements, such as sustainable materials and energy-efficient technologies, might be more expensive. Long-term rewards and savings, however, may be able to cover these expenses.

- **Budget Constraints:** When implementing green features, homeowners may have financial limitations. As such, it's critical to prioritise investments and look into low-cost options.

4.2. Materials and Expertise Availability

- **Material Accessibility:** Sustainable building materials could be more expensive or harder to get in some areas. It can be necessary for homeowners to look into other possibilities or collaborate with vendors that specialise in eco-friendly goods.

- **Skilled Professionals:** It can be difficult to locate designers and contractors with knowledge in green home design. To make sure they work with experienced specialists, homeowners might need to devote some time to study and screening.

4.3. Matters Concerning Regulation and Permits

- Building Codes and Regulations: Depending on the area, designing a green home may need adhering to a number of intricate building codes and regulations. Achieving the required permissions and making sure local codes are followed are essential for a successful deployment.

- Incentive Programs: Regional differences may exist in the availability and eligibility of rebates and incentives for green buildings. Homeowners who want to benefit from financial assistance can look into regional initiatives and incentives.

Green house design is a progressive method of building eco-friendly, effective, and hygienic living environments. Homes can lessen their influence on the environment, save money on utilities, and improve their general well-being by implementing the concepts of energy efficiency, resource conservation, and indoor environmental quality.

The advantages of designing a green home greatly exceed the drawbacks, which include upfront expenses, material availability, and regulatory concerns. Green home design is becoming increasingly feasible and accessible for homeowners worldwide thanks to sustained technological developments, rising environmental consciousness, and pro-environment legislation.

People who embrace green home design can benefit from the efficiency, comfort, and health advantages of an eco-friendly, well-designed home while also helping to create a more sustainable future.

➢ Energy-Efficient Home Design: Building Sustainable and Economical Structures

A key component of green home design is energy efficiency, which focuses on reducing energy use while preserving comfort and usefulness. Energy-efficient design improves indoor comfort, lowers utility costs, and lessens a home's total environmental effect. This article examines typical problems and their fixes, as well as the ideas and methods for creating energy-efficient homes and their advantages.

1. Energy-Efficient Home Design Principles

1.1. Structure Enclosure

- **Insulation:** An essential component of energy efficiency is adequate insulation. Reducing heat transfer through walls, ceilings, and floors keeps dwellings warmer in the winter and colder in the summer. Typical insulation materials consist of spray foam, cellulose, and fibreglass.

- Windows and Doors: Reducing heat gain and loss is greatly aided by energy-efficient windows and doors. Thermal performance can be enhanced via airtight sealing, low-emissivity (Low-E) coatings, and double or triple glazing. Drafts and heat loss can also be avoided with well-installed, insulated doors and windows.

1.2. Design and Orientation

- Passive Solar Design: By maximising natural sunshine for lighting and heating while minimising heat gain during warmer months, passive solar design concepts can be used. This entails planning the house so that windows facing southward will let in natural light, utilising thermal mass materials to retain and release heat, and adding shade elements like pergolas and overhangs.

- **Building Shape and Size:** A home's energy efficiency may be impacted by its size and shape. Heat gain and loss are minimised by compact, well-proportioned designs with little external surface area. Straightforward, rectangular designs are frequently more energy-efficient than intricate ones with plenty of angles and projections.

1.3. Systems that Use Less Energy

- **Heating, Ventilation, and Air Conditioning (HVAC):** Energy-efficient HVAC systems, like heat pumps, air conditioners, and high-efficiency furnaces, minimise energy usage without sacrificing comfort. By concentrating on particular rooms of the house, zoned heating and cooling systems can also maximise energy use.

- **Water Heating:** By heating water on demand or by drawing heat from the earth or air, energy-efficient water heating systems, such as tankless water heaters and heat pump water heaters, consume less energy. Another way to use renewable energy is using solar water heaters.

2. Methods for Putting Energy-Efficient Design into Practice

2.1. Lighting with Low Energy Use

- **LED Lighting:** Compared to conventional incandescent bulbs, LED bulbs can save up to 90% on energy consumption. Additionally, they last longer, which lowers waste and the need for replacements more frequently.

- **Lighting Controls:** By making sure lights are only turned on when necessary, installing lighting controls—such as dimmers, timers, and motion sensors—helps lower energy consumption.

2.2. Appliances with Low Energy Usage

- **Appliance Selection:** Selecting Energy Star-rated appliances guarantees that they adhere to strict guidelines for energy efficiency. This includes water-

and energy-efficient washing machines, refrigerators, dishwashers, and other home equipment.

- **Smart Appliances:** With advanced features like remote control, scheduling, and real-time monitoring, smart appliances help optimise energy use. These functions aid in more efficient energy management.

2.3. Integration of Renewable Energy

- **Solar Panels:** Photovoltaic (PV) solar panels installed on a home can produce clean, renewable energy. In addition to lowering dependency on the grid, solar panels can result in considerable long-term electricity cost savings.

- **Wind Turbines:** In locations with sufficient wind resources, small-scale wind turbines can produce power. They can be used in conjunction with solar power systems and offer an extra green energy source.

2.4. Technology for Smart Homes

- **Energy Management Systems:** These smart home technologies keep an eye on and regulate how much energy is used inside the house. They give homeowners access to real-time energy use data and let them change settings to maximise efficiency.

- **Smart Thermostats:** These devices adapt the heating and cooling settings based on user preferences that they learn. They have features like weather-based modifications and geofencing that can be configured remotely.

3. Advantages of Designing with Energy Efficiency

3.1. The Effect on the Environment

- **Reduced Carbon Footprint:** By using less energy, energy-efficient homes emit less greenhouse gases. This encourages a cleaner environment and aids in the battle against climate change.

- **Resource Conservation:** Making efficient use of water and energy lowers the pressure on water supplies and energy grids while also contributing to the conservation of natural resources.

3.2. Benefits to the Economy

- **Lower Utility Bills:** By consuming less energy, energy-efficient designs result in lower utility bills. Cost savings from lower heating, cooling, and lighting expenses can cover the upfront cost of energy-efficient equipment.

- **Increased Property Value:** Due to their lower operating costs and positive environmental effects, homes with energy-efficient features frequently fetch a higher price when they are put up for sale. This could be a big plus when it comes time to sell the house.

3.3. Increased Cosiness

- **Steady interior Climate:** By minimising drafts and temperature swings, energy-efficient designs contribute to the maintenance of a steady interior climate. This improves liveability and comfort levels all around.

- **Improved Indoor Air Quality:** By lowering moisture, pollutants, and allergens, effective ventilation, insulation, and HVAC systems help to improve indoor air quality.

4. Energy-Efficient Design: Challenges and Solutions

4.1. Start-Up Expenses

- **Upfront Investment:** Compared to more conventional solutions, installing energy-efficient design elements like windows, HVAC systems, and high-performance insulation may cost more. Long-term rewards and savings, however, can somewhat offset these upfront expenses.

- **Financing alternatives:** Homeowners can defray the upfront costs of energy-efficient modifications with the assistance of a variety of financing alternatives, including green building loans and energy-efficient mortgages.

4.2. Conceptualisation and Execution

- **Complex Design Considerations:** Orientation, materials, and systems are only a few of the many variables that must be carefully taken into account when designing for energy efficiency. Effective integration of energy-efficient techniques can be ensured by collaborating with skilled architects and builders.

- **Integration Challenges:** It could be necessary to make changes to the infrastructure or designs in order to include energy-efficient technology and systems. These obstacles can be overcome with careful preparation and expert assistance.

4.3. Upkeep & Maintenance

- **Continuous Maintenance:** To guarantee peak performance, energy-efficient systems and technologies need to have regular maintenance. To maintain systems in excellent working order, homeowners should arrange for routine maintenance and inspections.

- **System Upgrades:** As technology develops, new, more effective options can become available. For even greater energy efficiency, homeowners should stay up to date on new developments in technology and think about making improvements.

A crucial element of building affordable and sustainable homes is energy-efficient design. Homeowners can drastically lower their energy use and environmental effect by concentrating on ideas like building envelope optimisation, employing energy-efficient devices, and integrating renewable energy sources.

Beyond just saving money, energy-efficient design also improves interior air quality, increases comfort, and leaves a smaller carbon imprint. Even if there may be difficulties with initial prices and design complexity, these problems can be solved with the use of financing choices, expert advice, and continuing maintenance.

Energy-efficient house design will be essential in creating a more sustainable future as we continue to address environmental issues and look for solutions to lessen our impact on the environment. Adopting energy-efficient practices improves homeowners' and communities' quality of life in addition to making a positive impact on the environment.

➢ Eco-Friendly Home Renovation Tips: Using Sustainable Practices to Transform Your Space

During a home renovation, you have a great chance to incorporate eco-friendly choices and sustainable practices that improve your living space and the environment. Energy efficiency, resource conservation, and environmental impact reduction are the main goals of sustainable home remodelling. From planning and material selection to construction and post-remodelling considerations, this guide offers helpful advice for launching a sustainable renovation project.

1. Making a Renovation Plan

1.1. Establish Durable Objectives

- **Identify Priorities:** Choose the parts of remodelling your home that are most important to you, such as water saving, energy efficiency, or utilising sustainable materials. Establishing specific objectives makes decision-making easier and guarantees that sustainability will be a top priority for the duration of the restoration.

- **Assess Current Situations:** Examine your home's present state and pinpoint the areas that stand to benefit the most from renovations. Modernising windows or insulation, for instance, can significantly increase energy efficiency.

1.2. Budget and Research

- Research Sustainable techniques: Learn about the technologies and techniques of sustainable remodelling. Make educated judgements by learning about eco-friendly design concepts, low-impact materials, and energy-efficient technologies.

- Establish a Reasonable Budget: Create a budget that takes into consideration the upfront expenses as well as the long-term savings related to environmentally friendly remodelling. Take into account prospective power bill savings, rising property values, and any possible rebates or incentives.

2. Choosing Eco-Friendly Materials

2.1. Sustainable Construction Materials

- Recycled and Reclaimed Materials: Select materials that have been recycled or reclaimed to cut down on waste and the need for fresh resources. Repurposed bricks, recycled glass tiles, and salvaged timber are a few examples.

- Sustainable Sourcing: Choose materials like bamboo, cork, or quickly renewable fibres that are supplied sustainably. When compared to conventional choices, these materials have a lesser environmental impact.

2.2. Finishes that are Non-Toxic and Low-VOC

- Low-VOC Paints: To lessen indoor air pollution and promote a healthier living environment, choose low-VOC (volatile organic compound) paints and finishes. These paints have less of an effect on indoor air quality and emit less hazardous compounds.

- Non-Toxic Sealants: To prevent exposure to hazardous substances, use non-toxic sealants and adhesives. Seek out goods that emit little or no emissions to guarantee a safer environment inside.

3. Enhancing Energy Effectiveness

3.1. Air sealing and insulation

- Upgrade Insulation: Make an investment in high-performing materials for the floors, walls, and ceilings. Better insulation lowers heating and cooling expenses while assisting in the maintenance of a comfortable interior temperature.

- Seal Gaps and Leaks: To stop drafts and heat loss, locate and seal any gaps, cracks, and leaks around windows, doors, and other openings. Appropriate air sealing lowers the burden on heating and cooling systems and improves energy efficiency.

3.2. Systems That Use Less Energy

- Install Energy-Efficient Appliances: Swap out outdated appliances with ENERGY STAR-certified energy-efficient models. These appliances can drastically lower utility expenses because they use less energy.

- **Upgrade HVAC Systems:** If your home needs heating, ventilation, and air conditioning (HVAC), think about switching to a high-efficiency system. High-efficiency furnaces and heat pumps are two examples of options that can reduce energy use and increase comfort.

4. Strategies for Conserving Water

4.1. Fixtures with Low Flow

- **Install Low-Flow Showerheads and Faucets:** These fixtures use less water without compromising on functionality. They reduce utility costs and aid with water conservation.

- **Upgrade Toilets:** Water-efficient toilets that require less water to flush should be installed. Low-flow or dual-flush models are good choices for cutting back on water usage.

4.2. Harvesting Rainwater

- **Collect Rainwater:** To gather and store rainwater for irrigation and other non-potable needs, install a rainwater harvesting system. This promotes sustainable landscaping techniques and lessens dependency on municipal water supply.

5. Improving the Quality of Indoor Environment

5.1. Lighting and Natural Ventilation

- **Maximise Natural Ventilation:** Include vents, movable windows, and skylights in your remodelling design to improve natural ventilation. Enough ventilation lowers the demand for mechanical cooling while also improving the quality of the air indoors.

- **Utilise Natural Light:** Installing larger windows, skylights, or light tubes will increase the amount of natural light used. A setting with natural lighting is more comfortable to live in and requires less artificial lighting.

5.2. Air Quality Indoors

- **Select Low-Toxicity Materials:** To enhance indoor air quality, use finishes and materials with low levels of emissions and toxins. Steer clear of products that release hazardous chemicals or volatile organic compounds (VOCs).

- **Incorporate Plants:** By removing pollutants and raising oxygen levels, indoor plants can improve air quality. Select non-toxic, low-maintenance plants to create a healthier home atmosphere.

6. Eco-Friendly Building Techniques

6.1. Minimising Waste

Minimise Construction Waste: Make plans to recycle construction trash, donate useable goods, and reuse supplies in order to reduce waste during the remodelling process. Putting waste reduction strategies into practice lessens the project's negative environmental effects.

- **Select a Green Contractor:** Assist a contractor with knowledge of environmentally friendly building techniques. Making sure your refurbishment complies with eco-friendly guidelines and practices might be facilitated by hiring a green contractor.

6.2. Techniques for Energy-Efficient Construction

- **Incorporate Energy-Efficient Techniques:** Make use of building methods that improve energy efficiency, such using energy-efficient windows and doors or building with passive solar design principles.

- **Observe Construction Methods:** Make sure your building methods support your sustainability objectives. Verify on a regular basis that environmentally friendly construction methods are followed and that materials are handled responsibly.

7. Considerations After Renovation

7.1. Inspection and Upkeep

- **Monitor Performance:** To make sure energy-efficient systems and materials are operating as intended, keep an eye on their performance once your renovation is complete. Monitor water and energy use to see how well your changes are working.

- **Regular Maintenance:** To keep appliances and systems operating well, do routine maintenance. This includes doing insulation inspections, filter cleanings, and HVAC system maintenance.

7.2. Evaluate and Modify

- **Evaluate Outcomes:** Determine how your refurbishment will affect water and energy usage as well as sustainability in general. If necessary, use this information to make additional tweaks or changes.

- **Remain Updated:** Stay abreast with developments in environmentally friendly technologies and methods.

When new items and solutions emerge, think about implementing them in upcoming remodelling projects.

Numerous advantages come with renovating a home sustainably, such as less of an impact on the environment, less utility bills, and better interior air quality. Through adherence to these guidelines and an emphasis on energy efficiency, water conservation, and environmentally friendly materials, homeowners may convert their spaces into more comfortable and sustainable settings.

Although there may be early expenses and material availability issues, they may be addressed with careful planning, study, and working with experienced professionals. Adopting sustainable renovation techniques improves your home's overall quality of life while simultaneously making a positive impact on the environment.

Chapter 10

Living Sustainably Beyond the Home

Living sustainably involves much more than just staying in one's house. It includes a wholistic perspective on our interactions with the environment, impacting our decisions about consumption, mobility, and community engagement. Adopting sustainable methods in all facets of life encourages resource conservation, a more thoughtful way of living, and a healthier planet. This book examines doable methods for leading a sustainable lifestyle outside the house, including community involvement, responsible consumption, and mobility.

1. Ecological Mobility

1.1. Less Dependence on Automobiles

- **Public Transit:** By reducing the number of automobiles on the road, using public transport systems like buses, trains and subways helps lower individual carbon footprints. Compared to private vehicles, public transport is frequently more environmentally and energy-friendly.

- **Carpooling and Ride-Sharing:** Reducing the number of vehicles required for travel can be achieved by carpooling with others or by using ride-sharing services. This reduces emissions and traffic congestion. Having a sense of community is also enhanced by carpooling with neighbours or coworkers.

1.2. Other Modes of Transportation

- **Cycling**: Bicycling is a healthy, emission-free, and environmentally friendly form of transportation. Biking is becoming a more popular way to commute, and many cities have created bike lanes and bike-sharing programs to encourage it.

- **Walking:** Walking is the most environmentally friendly mode of transportation for short distances. It improves physical wellness, uses no fuel, and lowers pollution. Creating a walkable lifestyle, such as relocating close to a place of employment or other important services, can improve general wellbeing.

1.3. Vehicles that are Hybrid or Electric

- **Electric Vehicles (EVs):** EVs run entirely on electricity, which can come from renewable sources, and emit no tailpipe emissions. There are frequently incentives and rebates offered to promote the use of electric vehicles.

- **Hybrid Vehicles:** Compared to conventional vehicles, hybrid automobiles offer better fuel economy and lower emissions by combining electric propulsion with internal combustion engines. If you're making the switch to more environmentally friendly transportation, they might be a useful choice.

2. Conscientious Use

2.1. Selecting Sustainable Foods

- Local and Seasonal Foods: Supporting local farmers and reducing transportation-related carbon emissions are two benefits of buying locally grown and seasonal foods. Fresh, local vegetables can be found in plenty through community-supported agriculture (CSA) initiatives and farmers' markets.

Reduced intake of meat and dairy products can help reduce greenhouse gas emissions and the environmental effect of food production in **plant-based diets**. Increasing the amount of plant-based foods in your diet promotes sustainability in general.

2.2. Minimising Plastics with Single Use

- Reusable Alternatives: Use reusable products like shopping bags, food containers, and water bottles in favour of single-use plastics. This easy change minimises pollution to the environment and cuts down on plastic trash.

- **Products Without Plastic:** Select goods that come in little or no plastic packaging. Choose products that come in cardboard, metal, or glass packaging, and give firms that value eco-friendly packaging a boost.

2.3. Green Purchasing

- **Ethical Brands:** Promote businesses that show a dedication to environmentally friendly products, ethical labour standards, and waste minimisation. Make sure products and companies fit your ideals by doing some research on them.

- **Minimalist Perspective:** Embrace a minimalist approach and prioritise quality over quantity. Purchase only what you require, giving priority to sturdy, long-lasting goods that cut down on waste and the number of replacements needed.

3. Engagement with the Community

3.1. Encouragement of Local Projects

Participate in neighbourhood sustainability projects, such as recycling campaigns, clean-up days, and community gardens. Taking part in these initiatives promotes a feeling of community responsibility and helps to improve local settings.

- **Local Businesses:** Give locally owned companies and craftspeople a boost when it comes to sustainable practices. Buying locally boosts the local economy and lowers emissions from transportation.

3.2. Education and Advocacy

- **Environmental Advocacy:** Promote national, regional, and local environmental laws and regulations. Become involved with or lend assistance to organisations that address issues of sustainable development, conservation, and climate change.

- **Educational Outreach:** Use seminars, social media, or neighbourhood gatherings to educate others about sustainability. Teaching people about environmentally friendly behaviours promotes awareness and the wider acceptance of sustainable lifestyles.

3.3. Activism and Volunteering

- Volunteer Opportunities: Offer your assistance to groups that prioritise social justice, sustainability, or environmental preservation. In addition to offering practical experience, volunteering has a significant impact on ecosystems and communities.

- Activist Engagement: Take part in campaigns, demonstrations, or advocacy work to bring attention to environmental problems and advance sustainability. Activism increases public awareness of important environmental issues and promotes systemic change.

4. Innovation and Sustainable Technology

4.1. Eco-Friendly Technology

- **Energy-efficient Gadgets:** Try incorporating solar-powered chargers or smart home appliances that maximise energy usage into your everyday routine. These developments lessen their influence on the environment and energy consumption.

- **Sustainable Design:** Encourage the use of technologies that put an emphasis on sustainable design concepts, such as energy-efficient operation, recyclable materials, and low-impact manufacturing techniques.

4.2. Encouragement of Innovation

- **Research and Development:** Keep up with developments in environmentally friendly technology and lend your support to studies and projects that try to find novel ways to solve environmental problems.

- **Crowdfunding and Investment:** Take into account lending a hand to environmentally conscious businesses and initiatives via investments or crowdfunding websites. Your assistance can spur good change and help introduce cutting-edge, environmentally friendly solutions to the market.

5. Conscientious Lifestyle and Consumption

5.1. Mindful Consumption

- Thoughtful Purchases: Choose the goods and services you use with knowledge. Consider the effects that your purchases will have on society and the environment before making decisions that support your sustainability objectives.

- Reduce, Reuse, Recycle: Adhere to the maxims of cutting waste, recycling materials, and reusing products. You may lessen your influence on the environment and promote a circular economy by implementing these principles into your daily life.

5.2. Individual Welfare

- **Physical and Mental Health:** Adopt a sustainable way of living that enhances both physical and mental health. Take part in stress-relieving, nature-focused, and health-promoting activities, such as outdoor exercise, mindfulness training, and a balanced diet.

- **Work-existence Balance:** Make an effort to lead a balanced existence that is consistent with your beliefs about sustainability. Seek methods to incorporate environmentally friendly behaviours into your professional and personal life, and give top priority to pursuits that support a happy and sustainable living.

Living sustainably extends outside the house and requires a holistic approach to all aspects of everyday life, from consumption and transportation to community service and technological innovation. Through implementing environmentally conscious behaviours in every aspect of their lives, people may promote a more conscientious and conscientious way of living, lessen their impact on the environment, and keep the planet healthy.

Making deliberate decisions, staying informed, and being dedicated to making positive changes are all necessary for adopting a sustainable lifestyle. We can all work together to create a more sustainable future for ourselves and future generations by supporting neighbourhood projects, making ethical decisions, and keeping up with sustainability developments.

➢ Eco-Friendly Transportation

Degradation of the environment and greenhouse gas emissions are largely caused by transportation. Our travel habits are a major source of pollution and have a significant effect on the environment. Choosing environmentally friendly modes of transportation can help you save money, protect the environment, and lessen your carbon footprint. This book examines a range of tactics and options for implementing more environmentally friendly driving habits, such as switching to alternative fuel cars or altering one's lifestyle to commute more sustainably.

1. Using Vehicles with Alternative Fuels

1.1. EVs, or Electric Cars

- Overview: Electric vehicles emit no tailpipe emissions since they run on electricity rather than petrol or diesel. They are a great option to lessen dependency on fossil fuels and air pollution.

- Benefits: Electric vehicles (EVs) have a number of advantages over internal combustion engines (ICEs), such as reduced maintenance costs, quieter operation, and fewer moving parts. To promote the use of electric vehicles, several countries provide rebates or tax credits.

- Charging Infrastructure: The network of public charging stations expands together with the popularity of electric vehicles. Nowadays, a lot more homes and businesses have EV chargers, and improvements in fast-charging technology are enabling EV users to go farther between charges.

1.2. Hybrid Cars

- Overview: A hybrid car combines an electric motor and internal combustion engine. They minimise pollution and increase fuel efficiency by using the gasoline engine at higher speeds and the electric motor at lower ones.

- Benefits: Hybrid vehicles are less harmful to the environment overall and have better fuel efficiency than conventional gasoline-powered vehicles. Regenerative braking, which gathers and stores energy that would otherwise be lost, is another advantage for them.

1.3. Vehicles Using Hydrogen Fuel Cells

- Overview: Hydrogen fuel cell vehicles produce only water vapour as a byproduct of the chemical interaction between hydrogen and oxygen, which produces energy.

They provide a zero-emission substitute for traditional automobiles.

- **Benefits:** Compared to battery electric vehicles, hydrogen fuel cells offer longer driving ranges and quicker refuelling times. The lack of hydrogen refuelling stations in current use, however, can make widespread adoption difficult.

2. Encouragement of Public Transport

2.1. The Advantages of Public Transportation

- **Reduced Emissions:** Compared to private vehicle travel, public transport systems like buses, trains, and subways are more efficient, resulting in lower emissions per person and less traffic congestion overall.

- **Cost Savings:** Compared to buying and maintaining a personal vehicle, using public transport can be more economical. For frequent riders, several cities provide inexpensive passes or fee discounts.

2.2. Improving Transportation Networks

- Infrastructure Investment: Increasing accessibility, increasing frequency, and extending routes are just a few ways to improve public transportation's infrastructure and attract more riders.

- Integration with Other Modes: Creating integrated transportation networks that link public transportation to other forms of transportation, such ride-hailing services and bike-sharing schemes, can enhance general convenience and efficiency.

3. Encouragement of Walking and Cycling

3.1. Cycling's Advantages

- Environmental Impact: Cycling lessens dependency on motor vehicles and emits no pollutants. It also promotes cleaner urban areas and lessens transportation congestion.

- **Health Benefits:** Cycling is a great kind of activity that improves general health and physical fitness. It can also lessen stress and enhance mental health.

3.2. Encouraging Footwear

- **Short-Distance Travel:** For many daily errands, walking can be a car substitute for short excursions. It lessens the demand for transportation that relies on fossil fuels and encourages a more active lifestyle.

- **Urban Planning:** Creating walkable neighbourhoods with green areas, safe pedestrian routes, and easily accessible facilities promotes walking as a practical mode of transportation.

3.3. Building Infrastructure for Cycling

- **Bike Lanes and Racks:** Designating specific bike lanes and erecting bike racks in strategic places can improve cycling's convenience and safety. Infrastructure improvements for cyclists promote an active transportation culture.

- Bike-Sharing Programs: By allowing people to hire bicycles for short trips, bike-sharing programs help people commute more sustainably and decrease the need for private vehicles.

4. Introducing Ride-Sharing and Carpooling

4.1. The Advantages of Carpooling

- Decreased Emissions: By reducing the number of cars on the road, carpooling helps to lower total emissions as well as traffic congestion. Splitting the cost of transportation with others also reduces fuel use.

- Cost Efficiency: Since participants split expenditures like gas and parking, carpooling can drastically reduce transportation costs.

4.2. Services for Ride-Sharing

- **Overview:** By offering on-demand transportation options, ride-sharing services like Uber and Lyft provide an alternative to traditional automobile ownership. These days, a lot of these businesses include eco-friendly auto options, such as electric and hybrid vehicles.

- **Benefits:** Ride-sharing can increase mobility flexibility and lessen the requirement for private vehicle ownership. It also provides the opportunity to lower emissions when driving hybrid or electric cars.

5. Examining Sustainable Options for Travel

5.1. Journey by Train

- **Benefits:** Trains are a particularly energy-efficient form of transportation when they run on renewable energy. They can be more comfortable for long-distance travel and have a lower carbon footprint than flying.

- **Considerations:** Train travel can be a practical and environmentally responsible substitute for driving or flying in areas with well-developed rail networks.

5.2. Ferries: Electric and Hybrid

- **Overview:** Electric and hybrid ferries are being introduced as environmentally friendly substitutes for conventional diesel-powered vessels in certain riverine and coastal areas. These ferries promote cleaner water transportation by lowering emissions.

- **Advantages:** Electric and hybrid ferries are a quieter, more effective form of transportation and help to lessen maritime pollution.

6. Developing an Attitude towards Sustainable Transportation

6.1. Modifications to Lifestyle

- **Telecommuting:** By adopting telecommuting or remote work, one can lessen the need for daily commuting, which will cut down on emissions and traffic jams. Remote work has been shown to be environmentally friendly and productive by many companies and employees.

- **Effective Route Planning:** Arrange errands in a way that minimises travel lengths and cuts down on the number of trips needed. Fuel consumption can be decreased and travel routes can be optimised with the use of GPS and route planning apps.

6.2. Increasing Conscience

- **Education and Advocacy:** Raise public understanding of how travel affects the environment and push for environmentally friendly transport options. More comprehensive change can be sparked by taking part in community projects and advocating for laws that promote environmentally friendly modes of transportation.

- **Personal Responsibility:** Motivate people to consider how they might lessen their carbon footprint and accept accountability for their transportation decisions. Making environmentally friendly choices yourself and by setting an example can encourage others to follow suit.

One essential element of a sustainable lifestyle is environmentally efficient transportation. People may greatly lessen their environmental impact and help create a cleaner, healthier world by adopting alternative fuel vehicles, using public transport, encouraging cycling and walking, and supporting ride-sharing. Sustainable transportation methods improve community connectivity, individual well-being, and the environment.

Adopting these tactics necessitates a dedication to making deliberate decisions and endorsing more extensive programs that advance environmentally friendly transportation. Adopting and supporting environmentally friendly transport solutions will be essential to creating a more sustainable future for everyone as infrastructure and technology continue to advance.

➢ Community Involvement and Advocacy

Advocacy and community involvement are crucial for promoting real change in the direction of sustainability. People and organisations can influence sustainable behaviours and cultivate a sustainability culture by actively engaging in local activities, supporting environmental causes, and pushing for sustainable policy. This manual examines community involvement and sustainability advocacy, emphasising doable tactics and real-world instances.

1. Taking Part in Regional Sustainability Projects

1.1. Social Initiatives

- **Community Gardens:** Grow fresh, local produce and encourage green spaces in your neighbourhood by starting or participating in a community garden. In addition to promoting local food production and improving food security, community gardens also offer educational opportunities on sustainable agriculture.

- **Clean-Up Events:** Take part in or plan neighbourhood clean-ups to combat pollution and rubbish in public areas. These gatherings promote environmental stewardship and trash reduction while also helping towns become more aesthetically pleasing and clean.

- **Recycling Programs:** To enhance resource recovery and trash management, support or promote neighbourhood recycling initiatives. Engage in neighbourhood recycling programs and inform people about appropriate recycling techniques.

1.2. Encouragement of Local Companies

- **Eco-Friendly Businesses:** Support neighbourhood establishments that put an emphasis on sustainable methods including utilising eco-friendly materials, cutting waste, and encouraging ethical labour practices. Your encouragement fuels consumer demand for goods and services that respect the environment.

- **Farmers' Markets:** Purchase things produced by regional farmers and craftsmen who use sustainable and locally sourced materials by going to farmers' markets. Farmers' markets foster ties within the community and lessen the carbon footprint involved with the transportation of food.

1.3. Opportunities for Volunteering

- **Environmental Organisations:** Participate in volunteer work with groups that prioritise social justice, sustainability, and environmental preservation. Opportunities could be in the form of environmental lobbying work, educational outreach, or habitat restoration.

- **Non-Profit Groups:** Numerous non-profit organisations focus on regional and international sustainability projects. Give these organisations your time and expertise to help them reach their objectives and improve the environment.

2. Promoting Sustainable Policy

2.1. Taking Part in Local Policy Development

- **Attend Public Meetings:** Show your support for sustainable policies and initiatives by attending town halls, city council meetings, and local government meetings. Encourage legislators and local authorities to support sustainability and environmental preservation.

- **Post Comments for the Public:** During public comment periods, provide your opinions on proposed projects or policies. Provide your thoughts on the potential environmental effects of the suggested activities, along with suggestions for enhancements or changes.

2.2. Encouragement of Environmental Law

- **Get in Touch with Elected Officials:** Speak with your legislators to show your support for sustainable policies and environmental laws. Encourage policies that protect natural resources, combat climate change, and advance renewable energy.

- **Lobbying and Campaign:** Participate in campaigns and lobbying activities in favour of particular environmental laws or causes. Participate in advocacy and grassroots organisations that seek to reform systems and sway policy decisions.

2.3. Increasing Conscience

- **Educational Outreach:** To increase public understanding of sustainability and environmental issues, host or take part in workshops, seminars, or other educational events. Distribute knowledge about issues including waste minimisation, energy conservation, and sustainable living.

- Social Media: Connect with people who share your interests in sustainability, share materials, and advocate for environmental causes using social media platforms. Social media can be an effective tool for raising awareness, distributing success stories, and organising support.

3. Establishing Eco-Friendly Communities

3.1. Promoting Teamwork

- Partnerships: Work together to create and carry out sustainability projects with neighbourhood companies, associations, and organisations. Partnerships can strengthen the effects of initiatives and establish a network of people who support environmental initiatives.

- **Involvement in the Community:** Engage locals in the decision-making process around sustainability initiatives. To guarantee that projects fit the requirements and interests of the community, get opinions and input from a variety of sources.

3.2. Promoting Ecological Behaviours

- **Green Building Initiatives:** Encourage or support the use of sustainable materials, water-saving techniques, and energy-efficient design in both new and existing structures. Encourage certifications and norms that honour ecologically conscious building practices.

- **Transport Alternatives:** Promote the use of environmentally friendly modes of transport like carpooling, cycling, and public transport. Encourage infrastructural upgrades that increase the accessibility and convenience of sustainable mobility.

3.3. Encouragement of Social Equity

- **Inclusive Initiatives:** Make sure that sustainability initiatives take social equality into account and benefit the entire community. Speak up in favour of laws and initiatives that advance environmental justice and lessen inequities in the opportunities and resources available to people.

- **Affordable Solutions:** Encourage programs that give low-income families and marginalised populations access to sustainable practices and technologies. Strive to create fair access to environmental advantages and remove obstacles to implementing eco-friendly solutions.

4. Effective Community Involvement Case Studies

4.1. Initiatives for Urban Farming

- **Example:** The "Detroit Black Community Food Security Network" encourages community gardening and urban farming in Detroit in order to build community resilience and supply fresh vegetables to underprivileged areas.

- **Impact:** The program has made healthier food more widely available, encouraged regional farming, and given locals the confidence to actively participate in their food systems.

4.2. Campaigns to Reduce Plastic Waste

- **Example:** The "Ban the Bag" campaign, which was started in a number of places, promotes the usage of reusable bags instead of single-use ones. Bans on plastic bags and heightened public awareness of plastic pollution are results of the campaign.

- **Impact:** The campaign has been successful in promoting reusable products, cutting down on plastic waste, and influencing local and regional legislative reforms.

4.3. Projects Using Renewable Energy

- **Example:** Communities can purchase and install solar panels at a reduced cost by working together through the "Solarise" program. The initiative has facilitated the community's adoption of renewable energy technologies and increased access to solar energy.

- **Impact:** The program has boosted solar energy usage, lowered energy expenses, and helped the community achieve its sustainability objectives.

Advocacy and community involvement are essential for promoting environmental change and a sustainable society. Individuals and organisations can make a significant contribution to the transition to a more sustainable future by actively engaging in neighbourhood projects, endorsing eco-friendly laws, and fighting for environmental justice. Participating in these initiatives helps the environment as well as fostering community ties and giving people the confidence to change the world for the better.

Together, we can address environmental issues, advance sustainability, and build resilient, environmentally friendly communities by acting as a group and advocating for these goals. By adopting these values and setting a positive example, you may encourage others to join the cause and help create a healthy planet for present and future generations.

Conclusion

Welcome to a Greener Future

As we come to a close of our investigation into eco-friendly house hacks, it is evident that sustainable living is a significant and essential change that is required to create a world that is healthier and more balanced, rather than just a passing fad. Going through this book has opened my eyes to a number of ways to improve your quality of life and turn your house into an environmental role model.

The Way to Live Sustainable

The ideas discussed in these chapters, which range from trash reduction to energy efficiency, highlight how crucial it is to incorporate eco-friendly behaviours into our everyday lives. Whether it's installing water-saving appliances, choosing sustainable materials, or installing energy-efficient appliances, each section has provided helpful guidance and doable actions that help create a greener house and a more sustainable future.

Solidarity for Change

The reforms that are being considered involve more than simply individual efforts; they also involve encouraging a sustainable culture across our communities. You may improve your own environmental impact and lead by example by incorporating eco-friendly habits like home composting, mindful consumption, and supporting renewable energy sources. Advocacy and community involvement are essential to boosting these initiatives because group activities can have more profound and long-lasting effects.

Difficulties and Possibilities

There are many chances along the way to having a greener home, but there are also obstacles to overcome. It takes perseverance and creativity to get beyond technological obstacles, handle privacy issues, and negotiate the challenges of sustainable house design. Every obstacle, meanwhile, also offers a chance for development and advancement. You may successfully overcome these challenges by embracing new technology, fighting for laws that will benefit them, and keeping up with the latest developments in sustainability.

A Request for Action

This book's ultimate objective is to motivate and enable you to make significant progress towards sustainable living. The information and resources offered are intended to allow you the self-assurance to make wise choices and carry out actions that uphold your moral principles and improve the world. Every little bit helps, and when combined, these little actions can have a significant positive impact on the environment.

Looking Forward

It's clear that the ideas of sustainability and environmentally friendly living will only grow as we move forward. The environment of green living will evolve as a result of policy changes, technological advancements, and increased awareness. You will be able to stay at the forefront of this important movement if you stay involved, keep learning, and adjust to new changes.

Finally, keep in mind that the transition to a more sustainable house and way of life is a continuous process. No matter how tiny a step you take, it adds up to a greater goal of environmental stewardship and a healthier earth. You can change your living environment and contribute to a more sustainable and just future for everyone by adopting these eco-friendly tips and supporting sustainable practices.

➢ Recap of Key Points

1. Overview of Sustainable Lifestyle

Importance of Sustainability: Stresses the necessity of implementing environmentally friendly behaviours in order to lessen negative effects on the environment and encourage a healthy planet.

Book Overview: Offers a thorough manual for increasing the sustainability of your house with useful advice and doable tactics.

2. Energy-related Efficiency

LED Lighting: Energy usage and utility costs are decreased when LED lights are used in place of incandescent bulbs.

Natural Light: Making the most of natural light helps save energy by lowering the demand for artificial lighting.

Programmable Thermostats: optimises the use of energy in the heating and cooling systems.

Insulation: Energy efficiency and heat loss are reduced by appropriate insulation.

Energy-Efficient Appliances: Selecting high-rated appliances lowers running expenses and overall energy usage.

3. Conserving Water

Low-Flow Fixtures: Water consumption can be decreased without compromising performance by installing low-flow showerheads and faucets.

Rainwater Harvesting: Municipal water resources are preserved by gathering and utilising rainwater for irrigation and other non-potable uses.

Efficient Irrigation Techniques: To reduce water wastage in gardening and landscaping, use drip irrigation and irrigate during cooler hours.

4. Eco-friendly Substances

Eco-Friendly Building Materials: Reclaimed wood, bamboo, and recycled metal are examples of sustainable materials that have a minimal negative influence on the environment.

Low-VOC Paints: Painting with paints that have a low volatile organic compound (VOC) content helps to protect the environment and improves indoor air quality.

Sustainable Furniture and Decor: Choosing furnishings composed of environmentally friendly materials and production techniques contributes to a greener house.

5. Reduction of Waste

Composting at Home: Composting organic waste produces nutrient-rich soil for gardening while lowering landfill contributions.

Recycling and Upcycling: By extending the life cycle of materials and upcycling objects, waste is decreased.

Reducing Single-Use Plastics: Cutting back on single-use plastics contributes to less waste and pollution in the environment.

6. Green Cleaning

DIY Natural Cleaning Solutions: Using natural materials in homemade cleaning solutions lessens the need for chemical-based products.

Reusable Cleaning Tools: When choosing reusable cleaning tools over disposable ones, waste is reduced.

Eco-Friendly Brands: Sustainability is promoted by endorsing companies who put an emphasis on environmental responsibility in their cleaning products.

7. Eco-Friendly Planting

Organic Gardening: Keeping soil and ecosystems healthier is possible by avoiding synthetic fertilisers and pesticides.

Native and Vertical Plants: By maximising available area and utilising native plants and vertical gardening methods, biodiversity is improved.

Water-Saving Gardening Tips: Water conservation and plant health are supported by implementing techniques like mulching and effective watering.

8. Consumption with Mind

Minimalism and Ethical Shopping: Choosing ethically and adopting a minimalist lifestyle lowers waste and promotes sustainable behaviours.

Advantages of Buying Second-Hand: Buying used goods lessens the need for new ones and has a smaller negative impact on the environment.

9. Renewable Energy Sources

Solar Panels and Wind Turbines: Putting in renewable energy systems, such as solar panels and wind turbines, decreases energy costs and lessens dependency on fossil fuels.

Geothermal Heating and Cooling: This economical and environmentally friendly energy source can be used for both heating and cooling purposes.

10. Designing Green Homes

Designing for Energy Efficiency: Energy consumption is decreased by incorporating design features that improve energy efficiency, such as high-performance windows and passive solar heating.

Sustainable Home Renovation Tips: Utilising recycled materials and energy-efficient upgrades, among other sustainable practices, throughout home renovations helps achieve environmental objectives.

11. Living Beyond the House in a Sustainable Way

Eco-Friendly Transportation**: Using public transportation, biking, walking, and other sustainable modes of transportation all help to lessen carbon footprint.

Community Involvement and Advocacy: Supporting environmental policies and taking part in neighbourhood sustainability projects fosters a wider range of community effects.

Embracing Change: The book exhorts readers to embrace environmentally friendly behaviours and make wise choices that enhance their personal wellbeing as well as the environment.

Ongoing Efforts: Every step taken in the direction of a more environmentally friendly way of living adds to a bigger picture of sustainability and environmental stewardship.

This summary provides a concise synopsis of the main ideas and helpful suggestions covered in the book, providing guidance on how to adopt eco-friendly habits and promote constructive change in your household and neighbourhood.

➢ Encouraging Continuous Improvement

Living sustainably is not a destination, but a continuous process. Embracing continual improvement is essential to accomplishing long-term environmental goals and adjusting to changing technology and solutions as you integrate eco-friendly activities in your community and home. Here's how to promote ongoing development in environmentally friendly living:

1. Keeping Knowledgeable and Well-Informed

1.1. Stay Up to Date with Trends

- **Read Articles and Research:** To stay informed about the most recent advancements and best practices, read articles, research papers, and reports on sustainability on a regular basis.

- **Sustain Industry Pioneers:** For information on the latest developments in sustainability, follow influential people in the industry and sign up for newsletters.

1.2. Take Part in Seminars and Workshops

- **Attend Educational Events:** Take part in conferences, seminars, and workshops that are centred around sustainability. These gatherings provide insightful information and chances to network with professionals and like-minded people.

- **Online Courses:** Participate in webinars and online courses covering a range of topics related to sustainable living, such as green building techniques and energy efficiency.

2. Assessing and Improving Procedures

2.1. Routine Evaluations

- **Perform House Inspections:** Evaluate your home's general sustainability, waste management strategies, and energy and water usage on a regular basis. Determine areas that need work and establish new objectives.

- **Monitor Development:** Maintain a record of your successes and difficulties as you use sustainable methods. Make use of this knowledge to hone your tactics and establish loftier goals.

2.2. Upgrade Materials and Technologies

- **Invest in New Technologies:** Keep up with cutting-edge developments in technology that can improve the sustainability of your house. Upgrade to stronger insulation, more modern renewable energy systems, or more energy-efficient appliances.

- **Adopt New Materials:** Investigate and employ more recent, environmentally friendly building supplies and materials as they become accessible. Make sure they fulfil your performance and environmental requirements.

3. Taking Part in Policy and Community Initiatives

3.1. Promote Change

- **Support Policy Initiatives:** Participate in regional and national campaigns to advance environmentally friendly laws and policies. Encourage projects that complement your objectives for sustainability.

- **Community Projects:** Take part in or start neighbourhood recycling programs, energy-saving campaigns, or green building projects, among other sustainability-focused community projects.

3.2. Collaborate with Others

- **Form Alliances:** Assist with neighbourhood businesses, associations, and organisations to jointly undertake sustainable projects. Initiatives can have a bigger impact and be more effective when they are supported by partnerships.

- **Share Knowledge:** Inform and inspire others to embrace environmentally friendly behaviours. Use local seminars, social media, or community meetings to share your experiences and views.

4. Putting Creativity and Innovation First

4.1. Test Novel Concepts

- **Appoint Novel Methods:** Have an open mind when experimenting with novel sustainable methods and tools. Try new things to get better results, whether it's a novel approach to recycle or a creative way to save water.

- **Creative Solutions:** To solve problems related to sustainability, be creative. Create and put into action fresh approaches that deal with particular problems in your household or neighbourhood.

4.2. Adjust to Input

- **Ask Input:** Ask your family, neighbours, and community members for input on your sustainability initiatives. Make changes and enhance your strategy with the help of this feedback.

- **Adapt and Evolve:** Be open to adjusting and adapting your methods in response to new knowledge, criticism, and evolving conditions. To be continuously improved, you have to be open to changing and improving your processes.

5. Highlighting Successes and Establishing New Objectives

5.1. Acknowledge Achievements

- **Celebrate Milestones:** Honour and commemorate the strides and victories you make towards a sustainable future. Acknowledging achievements promotes positive behaviour and keeps people motivated.

- **Share Success Stories:** Encourage and motivate others to follow similar habits by sharing your triumphs with them. Emphasising the advantages and favourable effects of sustainable living can promote its wider acceptance.

5.2. Set Ambitious Goals

- **Establish New aims.** Maintaining the momentum and pushing yourself further is facilitated by persistently posing challenges to yourself.

- **Make Future Plans:** Create a long-term sustainability plan that takes community involvement, continuing education, and future enhancements into account. Sustained success and advancement are guaranteed by a deliberate strategy.

Promoting sustainable living through constant improvement requires being informed, assessing and modernising methods, participating in community initiatives, welcoming innovation, and acknowledging accomplishments. By implementing these tactics, you may improve the efficiency of your sustainability initiatives, encourage constructive change in your household and neighbourhood, and help create a future that is more resilient and sustainable.

The pursuit of sustainability is a dynamic and continuous process, whereby every advancement made leads to the well-being of the earth. Adopting a continual improvement approach guarantees that your work is meaningful and relevant, promoting a sustainable culture that helps current and future generations.

www.ingramcontent.com/pod-product-compliance
Lightning Source LLC
Chambersburg PA
CBHW071910210526
45479CB00002B/353